Paediatric Radiology
for MRCPCH and FRCR
second edition

Dedication

This book is dedicated to our paediatric colleagues, who have tolerated our mistakes and enthused over our successes.

Paediatric Radiology
for MRCPCH and FRCR
second edition

Chris Schelvan
BSc MBBS MRCP FRCR
Consultant Radiologist & Honorary Senior Lecturer
Imperial College NHS Trust
St Mary's Hospital, London

Annabel Copeman
BSc MBBS FRCPCH
Consultant Paediatrician
Royal Wolverhampton Hospitals NHS Trust
Wolverhampton

Jacky Davis
MBBS FRCR
Consultant Radiologist
The Whittington Hospital, London

Annmarie Jeanes
MBBS MRCP FRCR
Consultant Paediatric Radiologist
Leeds Teaching Hospitals NHS Trust, Leeds

Jane Young
MSc MBBS FRCR
Consultant Radiologist
The Whittington Hospital, London

The ROYAL
SOCIETY *of*
MEDICINE
PRESS *Limited*

©2010 Royal Society of Medicine Press Ltd

Published by the Royal Society of Medicine Press Ltd
1 Wimpole Street, London W1G 0AE, UK
Tel: +44 (0)20 7290 2921
Fax: +44 (0)20 7290 2929
E-mail: publishing@rsmpress.ac.uk

British Library Cataloguing in Publication Data
A catalogue record for this book is available from the British Library

ISBN: 978-1-85315-702-8

Distribution in Europe and Rest of the World:
Marston Book Services Ltd
PO Box 269
Abingdon
Oxon OX14 4YN, UK
Tel: +44 (0)1235 465500
Fax: +44 (0)1235 465555
Email: direct.order@marston.co.uk

Distribution in USA and Canada:
Royal Society of Medicine Press Ltd
c/o BookMasters Inc
30 Amberwood Parkway
Ashland, OH 44805, USA
Tel: +1 800 247 6553/ +1 800 266 5564
Fax: +1 410 281 6883
Email: order@bookmasters.com

Distribution in Australia and New Zealand:
Elsevier Australia
30–52 Smidmore Street
Marrickville NSW 2204, Australia
Tel: +61 2 9517 8999
Fax: +61 2 9517 2249
Email: service@elsevier.com.au

Typeset by Phoenix Photosetting, Chatham, Kent
Printed by Bell and Bain Ltd, Glasgow

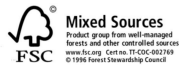

Contents

Foreword

Throughout my consultant career I have had two passions; my 'home' speciality of paediatric neurodisability, and the education of the next generation of doctors. Through my various education roles, initially as Director of Postgraduate Medical Education at Great Ormond Street Hospital, through Regional Adviser in Paediatrics for the RCPCH, to my most recent role as Head of School of Paediatrics for London, I have seen many changes in the delivery of clinical training. The two most significant changes have been firstly the move to a 'competency-based' model of training, and secondly the dramatic shortening of training time with the arrival of EWTD for junior doctors. These changes have had both positive and negative consequences – and when it comes to paediatric radiology, this book does much to offset the latter.

Those who have concerns about a competency-based approach to training worry that it can be reductionist – ensuring that certain standards are achieved, but at the same time risking a more rigid or mechanical approach to learning, rather than the more fluid approach that allowed trainees to follow their natural curiosity about the cases they encountered, and to acquire knowledge by a serendipitous process of self-directed discovery and adventure. Quite clearly, the two approaches are *not* mutually exclusive, and the huge advantage of this book is that it re-engenders the fun of puzzling over an X-ray or scan, learning about the key radiological points through the *radiology hot list* for each case, and then – very importantly – linking those to the relevant clinical 'pearls' or 'nuggets' through the *clinical hot list* sections. The authors point out that the book does not attempt to provide systematic coverage of the paediatric radiology curriculum, and thank heavens for that, because systematic can sometimes be rather dull! Rather the random sequence of the presented cases simulates real life, means that it's not a 'cover to cover' reading chore, and allows the reader to dip in and learn something important by working through a case or two on the train, in the lunch queue or indeed during any other 5 minute pit stop.

The other 'hot potato' in the medical press is the impact of shortened training on experiential or work-place based learning. In the past, trainees may have had the time in clinical practice to see many of the cases presented in this book in the flesh (or more accurately with the advent of PACS, in the pixels). Today, that is no longer achievable, so this collection of cases is the closest possible simulation of the sort of learning that regularly takes place on the ward round or in the radiology meeting. However, the accessible format packs in enough cases to simulate a great deal more wards rounds and radiology meetings than any trainee could possibly hope to attend.

Finally – although the authors have aimed this book at those on the more uncomfortable side of the MRCPCH and FRCR – it is important not to forget revalidation, and those of us on the other side of the fence. Personally I very much enjoyed a romp through the cases in the book, and I am sure that some older fossils like myself – particularly those who have entered a narrower subspeciality – will equally benefit from refreshing their general paediatrics in this way.

Two of the things that *have not* changed over the years is the enthusiasm of consultants for teaching and the appetite of trainees for learning. This book demonstrates the former and will surely feed the latter.

Hilary Cass
Neurodisability Consultant
Guy's and St Thomas' NHS Foundation Trust

Foreword from first edition

For the inexperienced (and sometimes experienced) doctor, dealings with children, radiological interpretation and the appropriate use of a wide range of imaging modalities are areas prone to pitfalls.

The interpretation of children's X-rays can be a daunting affair for both trainee paediatricians and radiologists, and the competences needed are acquired by reporting hundreds of routine, and not so routine, films. This book distils many radiological pearls of wisdom, wraps them in a familiar clinical scenario, and enables the trainee to absorb the important facts and first principles by which radiological diagnoses are made.

This book is orientated towards candidates for MRCPCH and FRCR. It aims to provide the trainee with diagnostic clues with which to improve their interpretation of paediatric imaging – but not just for the purpose of passing examinations. More importantly, it provides a framework to make a radiological diagnosis, or assist in a difficult diagnosis when presented with similar scenarios in the middle of the night.

Not so much a reference book, more a 'radiologist in your pocket' guide to paediatric radiology, equipping you for the rigours of examinations, and improving the care of patients. I would recommend that all trainees (and a few consultants) keep a copy near to hand.

Andrew Raffles
MBBS FRCPCH FRCP DCH
Consultant Paediatrician and Regional Advisor in Paediatrics to the
London Deanery
Queen Elizabeth II Hospital
E&N Herts NHS Trust
Welwyn Garden City, Herts

Preface

Radiology plays an important role in the diagnosis and management of childhood diseases. This is reflected in both paediatric and radiology postgraduate exams, where candidates are expected to have a working knowledge of paediatric pathology, clinical manifestations and appropriate radiological investigations.

The object of this book is twofold. Our primary aim is to get you through your exams! With this in mind, we have chosen examples of both important and common conditions that a paediatrician and a radiologist should be able to recognize, and in which the imaging findings are typical and diagnostic. Though primarily concentrating on plain radiographs, we have used all the different imaging modalities to encompass many of the paediatric radiology cases that a candidate is likely to encounter. Some of the cases included are rare in clinical practice, but frequently turn up in exams.

The cases are randomly ordered to reflect the nature of the exams. Each case includes key points about the radiological and clinico-pathological aspects of the condition – the 'hot lists'. In this way we have tried to distill out the essence of each condition to compliment the relative needs of a paediatrician and a radiologist in training.

The second objective is to give 'tools' in the form of methods for analyzing some types of imaging modalities. These can be used when you don't have access to a paediatric radiologist.

The first edition of this book was well received, and in view of this positive feedback we have kept the same format. However there have been significant advances in radiological technology in the last 7 years, with increasing use of and improved access to cross-sectional imaging, which is reflected in the new edition. New cases have been added, images have been updated and we have placed more emphasis on CT/MRI as these modalities become the bread-and-butter of radiological practice.

Radiation burden remains a significant worry in paediatric practice and there is an increasing awareness of non-accidental injury throughout society: we have added new sections to address these important areas.

This book does not aim to be a comprehensive guide to paediatric radiology – more of a whistle-stop-tour of classic films. We hope it helps you pass your exam!

Good luck!

Chris, Annabel, Jacky, Annmarie and Jane.

Acknowledgement

The authors would like to thank Dr Ranjana Chaudhuri of the Whittington Hospital, London, who provided some of the radiographs used in this book.

Rules and tools

Paediatric chest X-ray

HOW TO LOOK AT A PAEDIATRIC CHEST X-RAY

There is a lot of information on a chest X-ray (CXR) and it helps to have a routine. This takes less time than you think and avoids basic mistakes, for example assessing the wrong patient. You will also start to look at all the information present instead of just looking at the heart and lung fields.

1. **Elementary matters.** Check the name, date, side markers, and anything written on the film (e.g. 'film in expiration', 'lateral decubitus').
2. **Technical matters.** Ask yourself if the film is technically adequate. This sounds boring and unnecessary but this is why you must.

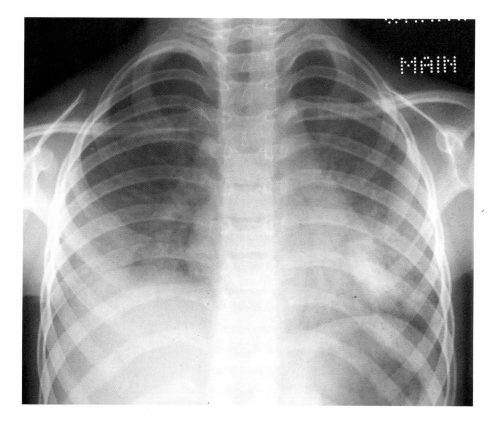

This child was admitted with a cough, and a chest X-ray (CXR) was performed. What does it show? What is the diagnosis?

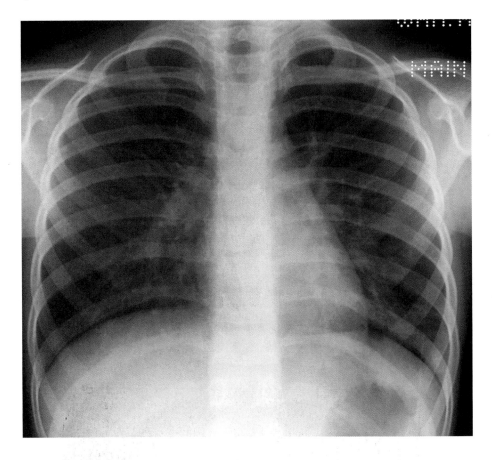

There is nothing the matter with the child's chest. The first film was taken in expiration (looking for air trapping). This film was taken immediately after the first one, and is in full inspiration. The lung fields are clear.

So you must assess the film for:

1. **Adequate inspiration**—five anterior ribs above the diaphragm.
2. **Rotation**—the medial ends of the clavicles should be equidistant from the spine.
3. **Penetration**—you should be able to see the spine through the heart.
4. **Lordotic projection**—this is usually due to the child arching away from the cassette. This can result in distortion of the superior mediastinum, and apparent upper lobe blood diversion along with a boot-shaped heart.

Now you can interpret the film

Make sure you include all of these in your review (you may find it helps if you leave the heart and lungs until last).

(1) Bones: including spine, ribs and proximal humeri

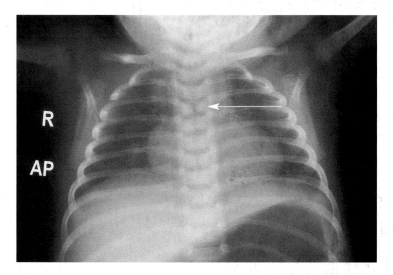

This child has a heart murmur: note the vertebral abnormality.

(2) Soft tissues

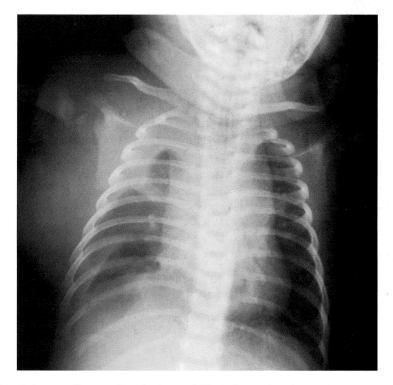

Note the soft tissue swelling over the right chest wall. This is due to a large haemangioma.

(3) Mediastinum including thymus

The thymus often causes difficulties in interpretation of the CXR because of its variable size and configuration. Typically it lies on both sides of the superior mediastinum and has a smooth lateral border. It blends inferiorly with the cardiac contour, although sometimes there is a little notch at the junction. It is of low density, and lung markings can usually be seen through it. The normal thymus does not displace the trachea or oesophagus. On the plain film it is usually apparent until the age of 2, although it may be seen in older children (up to 4 years and sometimes even older). The thymus may decrease in size in response to stress (e.g. infection) and return to normal when the child's clinical condition improves.

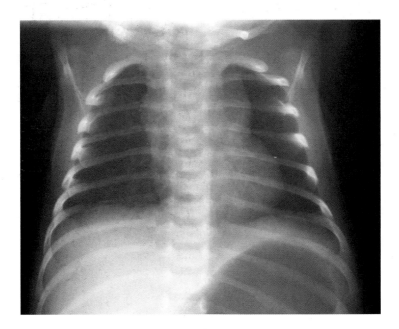

Typical appearance of the thymus.

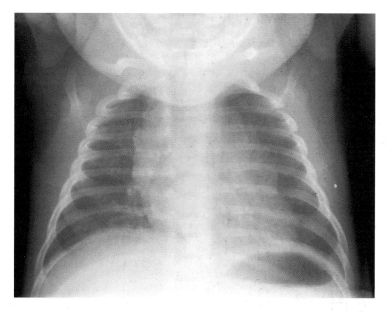

Typical appearance of the thymus.

(4) Heart

Assess the heart size but remember the film is usually taken anteroposterior (AP). In infants the thymic outline may give a false impression of cardiomegaly. Note the position of the aortic arch and assess the pulmonary vasculature (plethora/oligaemia).

(5) Lungs

- Check the lung volumes:
  — Overinflated? (e.g. bronchiolitis).
  — Asymmetrical? (e.g. inhaled foreign body).
- Focal pathology—mass, collapse, consolidation.
- Diffuse abnormality—fibrosis, oedema.

Review areas where you are likely to miss things. This should include:

1. **The superior mediastinum**—a difficult area, especially in younger children because of the presence of the thymus. Make sure you don't mistake the thymus for lymphadenopathy/consolidation (and vice versa).
2. **The hila**—check their position (are they displaced by lobar collapse?) and their size and density.
3. **Behind the heart**—look for left lower lobe collapse/consolidation and paravertebral pathology.
4. **Below the diaphragm**—remember children may have a lot of air in their stomach, particularly if they have been crying, or have just had a feed before the examination.

Note: The apices are an important review area in adults, but apical pathology is less common in children. An opacity projected over the apex is more likely to be a hair plait than a mass lesion.

Remember to check the position of tubes and lines.

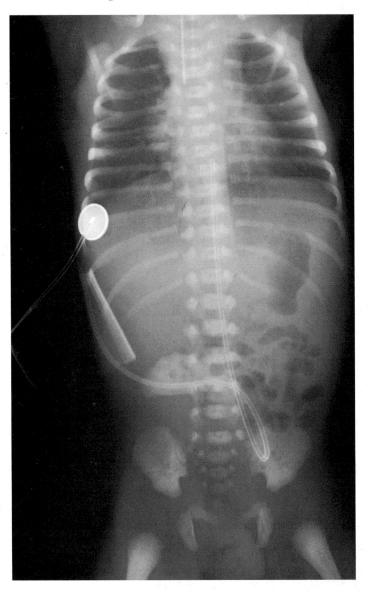

An umbilical artery catheter is present with its characteristic loop in the iliac artery in the pelvis. There is an endotracheal tube present.

Useful tips

1. Query any foreign body projected over the film—there is almost no small object that cannot be aspirated or swallowed.
2. Compare with previous films. Beware the child with many previous studies—they may have an underlying problem (e.g. cystic fibrosis), which has been overlooked.

Nuclear medicine

These are the scans that look like huge numbers of dots coalesced to form a blurred shape. It is however an excellent functional imaging modality used to assess the genitourinary, gastrointestinal, endocrine and musculoskeletal systems and is of vital importance in paediatric radiology.

RENAL NUCLEAR MEDICINE

This is the commonest type of paediatric nuclear medicine study performed in the district general hospital setting.

There are two types of renal scans:

1. **Static.** The tracer (DMSA) is taken up and retained by the kidney.
2. **Dynamic.** The tracer (MAG3 or DTPA) is taken up and excreted rapidly by the kidneys. Images of the renal tract are produced, and the passage of the tracer through the kidney is mapped by a graph, called a **renogram**.

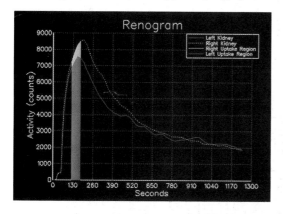

A normal renogram. The initial rise of the graph is the tracer arriving at the kidney through the bloodstream. The tracer then passes through the kidney, leading to the excretion (downward) part of the curve, when the tracer leaves the kidney in the urine.

In **obstruction**, the tracer accumulates in the collecting system and is not washed out.

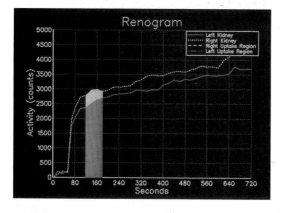

An obstructed renogram. The tracer arrives in the bloodstream (initial upward part of the graph). The graph continues to rise as tracer continues to arrive, but cannot leave the kidney.

Diuretics are necessary to confirm that this appearance is due to obstruction, rather than a 'baggy' slow-draining collecting system.

Nuclear cystogram

This is used in the detection of vesicoureteric reflux. The cystogram can be direct, when the tracer is introduced directly into the bladder, or indirect, performed at the end of the standard renogram (the voiding phase). A nuclear cystogram is preferred (where possible) to an X-ray cystogram as the radiation dose to the child is much less.

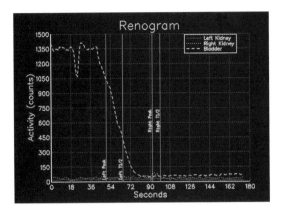

A normal cystogram. There is decreasing bladder activity during micturition, with no concurrent change in kidney activity.

An increase in the kidney activity during voiding indicates reflux. Sometimes this is evident even prior to voiding. A small 'blip' at the end of voiding is often seen when reflux is present as tracer returns to the bladder from the kidneys.

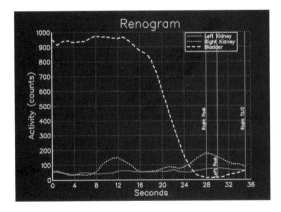

A cystogram showing vesicoureteric reflux. There is a concurrent rise in kidney activity during micturition as the bladder activity decreases.

STATIC SCANS

DMSA

This tracer is taken up by the renal parenchyma (proximal tubules). The study assesses functional renal tissue and is useful in assessment of:

- Differential renal function.
- Scarring secondary to a urinary tract infection (UTI). Defects are better demonstrated than on a renogram.
- Renal function in abnormal kidneys, for example multicystic dysplastic kidney and pelvi-ureteric junction (PUJ) obstruction.

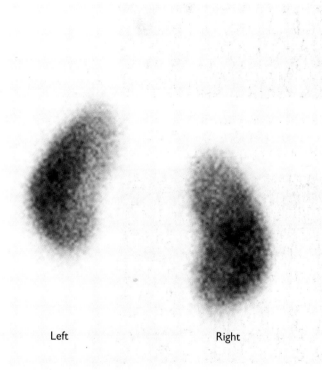

Left   Right

A normal DMSA scan. Note the reversed position of the kidneys due to posterior acquisition of the image.

Contrast studies

GASTROINTESTINAL STUDIES

Barium meal

- This is usually performed to assess the anatomy of the upper gastrointestinal (GI) tract and to exclude malrotation.
- Videofluoroscopy can be helpful in the investigation of children with feeding difficulties (e.g. assessment of swallowing and recurrent aspiration).

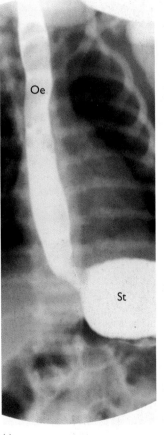
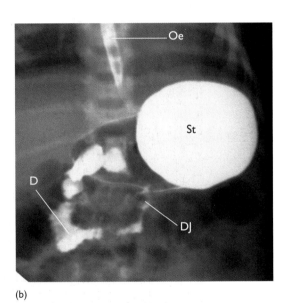

(a) (b)

(a, b) Normal barium meal showing oesophagus, stomach, duodenum and proximal jejunum. Oe = oesophagus, St = stomach, D = duodenum, DJ = DJ flexure, J = jejunum.

Large bowel studies (barium or water-soluble contrast)

- Can be therapeutic (e.g. meconium ileus) or diagnostic (e.g. atresias, microcolon), or both (intussusception).

INTRAVENOUS UROGRAM

Intravenous urograms (IVUs) are rarely performed, having been superceded by ultrasound, magnetic resonance urography (MRU) and CT urography (CTU).

MICTURATING CYSTOGRAM

This is performed to look for reflux and to assess the urethra in boys. Whether these are carried out under direct screening or as nuclear medicine studies will depend on local practice.

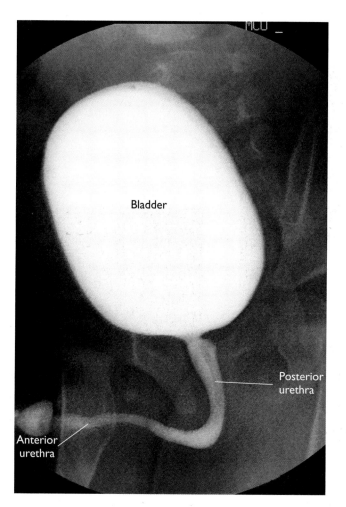

Normal cystogram in a boy.

Computed tomography

Computed tomography (CT) scans are exciting radiology investigations that produce plenty of exquisite anatomical pictures but at the cost of a very high radiation burden (request them with caution in children).

PHYSICS FOR DUMMIES

CT is essentially a glamorous X-ray machine, where both the X-ray beam and multiple detectors rotate around the patient in a spiral. X-rays shoot through the patient as the table moves continuously. A volume of radiological data is acquired, which can then be manipulated, so the images can be viewed in multiple planes with three-dimensional (3D) reconstructions. The classic CT image is a transverse image (an **axial slice**), but multi-detector CT allows the images to be viewed in any plane. Each image contains data that can be manipulated to look at bone, soft tissue, lungs, and brain (different windows).

Basic concepts

Appearance of lesion on CT (soft tissue windows)	CT number (density or attenuation)	Causes
White	High	Bone, calcification, acute haemorrhage, contrast agents (intravenous or oral)
Intermediate grey	Intermediate (between +100 and −20)	Water, soft tissue
Black	Low	Fat, air

But remember

The relative density of structures on CT depends on the window settings—the same structures will have completely different brightness levels on bone, lung and soft tissue windows.

ANATOMY FOR DUMMIES

We cannot teach you cross-sectional anatomy, but exams are all about 'classical pictures'—so learn to recognize normal anatomy on a few useful transverse anatomical levels.

Chest

- Normal appearances are shown in the figures below.
- Recognize the normal mediastinal contours and the position of normal vascular structures (aorta and its main branches, superior vena cava, pulmonary arteries).

(a)

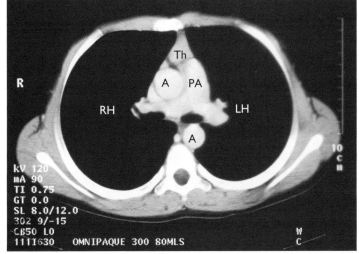

Contrast-enhanced CT chest at level of the hila. (a) Soft tissue windows. A = aorta, PA = pulmonary artery, RH = right hilum, LH = left hilum, Th = thymus.

(b)

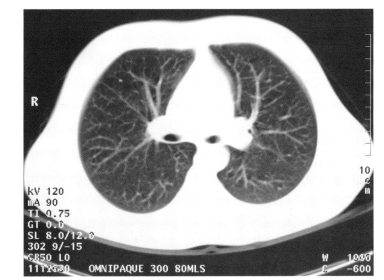

Contrast-enhanced CT chest at level of the hila. (b) Lung windows.

Abdomen

Normal appearances are shown below.

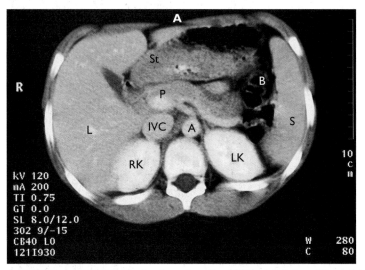

Contrast-enhanced CT of upper abdomen. L = liver, S = spleen, RK = right kidney, LK = left kidney, A = aorta, IVC = inferior vena cava, B = bowel, St = stomach, P = pancreas.

Brain

Normal CT appearances are shown below.

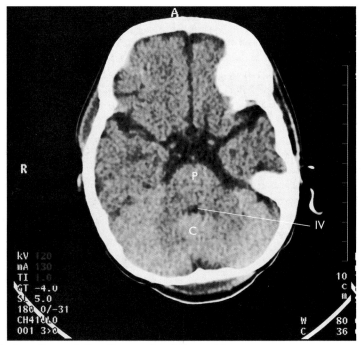

(a) Posterior fossa. C = cerebellum, P = pons, IV = IVth ventricle.

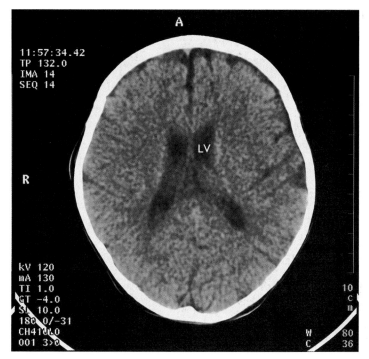

(b) Cerebral hemispheres. IV lateral ventricle.

Key points

- Be systematic—look at each organ in turn. Assess the size and look for irregularities in contour and density of each organ. If you are looking at paired or symmetrical structures (kidneys, adrenals, brain) compare the two sides.
- Has contrast been given? Look at the blood vessels, which will be bright.
- In the absence of contrast, soft tissue high density represents calcification or haemorrhage.
- In the chest, look for abnormal soft tissue in the mediastinum and lungs.
- In the abdomen look for abnormal soft tissue masses, free fluid and para-aortic lymphadenopathy.
- In the brain, look for midline shift and make sure the lateral ventricles are a normal size and symmetrical. Low-attenuation lesions may represent tumours, infarcts, or oedema. Do not forget to have a quick look at the sinuses and orbits. Bone windows are important in trauma cases.

Magnetic resonance imaging

Magnetic resonance imaging (MRI) is a sophisticated non-radiation imaging modality that may eventually become the bread-and-butter of radiology. It is particularly used for neuroradiology and musculoskeletal work, but has increasingly extensive applications in body imaging as well.

PHYSICS FOR DUMMIES

MRI uses non-ionizing magnetism instead of radiation. Different tissues contain different amounts of water (protons), so when a strong magnetic field is applied, the different tissues have different magnetic properties. This results in the exquisite soft tissue differentiation achieved with MRI.

T1 and T2 simply refer to different methods of sampling the magnetic resonance signal—meaning that the same soft tissue may have different signal characteristics on different sequences—for instance, fluid is low signal on T1 and high signal on T2.

The useful thing about MRI is that you can obtain images in any plane (the so-called 'multiplanar capacity' of MRI)—usually sagittal, coronal, or axial.

Key points

- **MRI** gives good soft tissue detail—useful in brain, spine and musculoskeletal work. There is no signal from bone—use CT to evaluate bone pathology.
- **Fluid** (and therefore oedema surrounding masses or within inflamed areas) appears low signal (dark) on T1 and high signal (white) on T2.
- **Gadolinium** (intravenous contrast) enhancement shows up as high-signal areas (white) on T1 scans (if it enhances it is usually pathological).

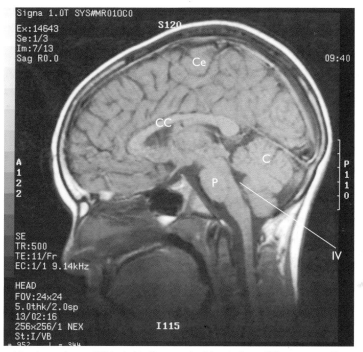

Sagittal T1-weighted scan (note: CSF is dark). Ce = cerebral hemisphere, CC = corpus callosum, P = pons, C = cerebellum, IV = IVth ventricle.

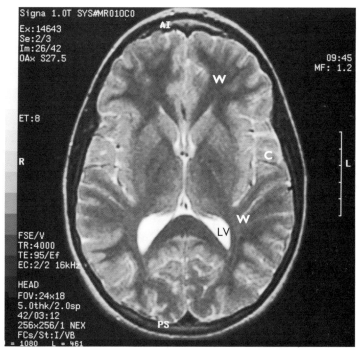

Axial T2-weighted scan at level of lateral ventricles (note: CSF is bright). C = cortex, W = white matter, LV = lateral ventricle.

Radiation protection and patient safety

Radiation is bad for you, and even worse for children.

The doses encountered in diagnostic imaging (or from background radiation exposure) result in potential cell damage. The risk of cell damage increases with duration and frequency of irradiation, and can potentially result in genetic mutations or neoplasia. This means that single low-dose exposures carry a much lower risk than multiple high-dose exposures.

Plain radiographs, fluoroscopy, CT and nuclear medicine imaging all involve some form of ionizing radiation, i.e. X-rays, gamma rays and beta particles. MRI does not involve ionizing radiation, using instead proton 'density' and magnetization characteristics of tissues. Ultrasound is one of the most frequently used imaging modalities in children because:

1. It involves no radiation, using soundwave technology.
2. It is relatively quick and portable.
3. Image quality is usually excellent, because children are smaller and generally have less body fat than adults.

The use of CT has risen exponentially over the past decade. The development of increasingly sophisticated equipment (multidetector technology) has allowed faster scanning times, 3D imaging and CT angiography, including cardiac scans. Unfortunately this improvement comes at the cost of a significantly increased radiation burden, which is most important in the paediatric population.

Whilst CT is limited by its substantial radiation burden, MRI has the advantage of being safe and radiation free. MRI remains limited by long scanning times—general anaesthesia may be required in young children, which limits its use.

The radiation delivered by specific investigations can be better judged by the equivalent number of chest X-ray exposures that would be required to match the radiation dose.

Estimated number CXR equivalents for varying investigations

Imaging modality	5-year-old child
Abdomen X-ray	15
Lumbar spine	30
CT brain	160
CT abdomen/pelvis	540
Micturating cysto-urethrogram (MCUG)	230
Barium meal	300
Bone scan	1560
USS	Nil
MRI	Nil

Selection of appropriate imaging investigation

The range of tests available increases year by year. Selection of a particular test depends on many factors. The availability, accuracy, radiation burden, degree of invasiveness and need for sedation/anaesthesia will all influence the choice.

Remember some general principles:

1. The more information you give a radiologist, the better the quality of report you get. Discussing a sick/worrying child with the radiologist usually helps both parties. They are the experts in imaging, so use them.
2. The chance of a test yielding a positive result increases if the clinical evidence of the condition is high (known as a high pretest probability).
3. Some tests are very good at confirming or excluding the diagnosis, for example ultrasound for a hip effusion (a sensitive and specific test). Some tests are very good at telling you if something is present (sensitive) but a negative result does not exclude the diagnosis (not specific), for example ultrasound in acute appendicitis.
4. It is important to be aware of the potential risks to the infant and young child when they are exposed to radiation—no radiation is good radiation!

Always try to keep radiation dose to a minimum or use a non-ionizing investigation first!

Non-accidental injury

Non-accidental injury (NAI) is deliberate abuse by a parent or guardian, and its true incidence is not known. Abuse is often occult and there may be few clinical signs. Abuse may be physical, emotional, sexual, involve neglect and fabricated or induced illness (FII, previously referred to as Munchausen by proxy). It is more often a mixture of all of these.

Paediatricians and radiologists play a vital role in ensuring child safety where there are concerns that a child may have suffered harm. There are a number of clinical indicators in the presentation, history, examination findings and/or family background that may lead to a request for imaging. Alternatively, the radiologist may detect suspicious fractures or other features when a child is imaged for unrelated reasons, thus triggering concerns about NAI.

Physical abuse may involve the brain and/or the skeletal system. Infants may suffer brain injury as a consequence of shaking or direct impact injuries. They may present with collapse, apnoeas, seizures or acute life-threatening events.

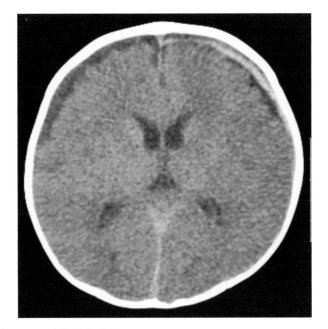

CT brain showing an acute left subdural haematoma.

Older children more commonly present with fractures, but brain injury may be occult in older age groups. After dealing with any acute injuries, a full skeletal survey and a head CT should be performed. The skeletal survey consists of a standard series of radiographs to visualize the whole skeleton. The purpose of this is to detect any occult skeletal injuries and to exclude any underlying skeletal disorders that may predispose to fractures, such as osteogenesis imperfecta. The CT of the brain is recommended to exclude occult intracranial injury.

Fractures are common in both accidents and abuse, and differentiating the two may be difficult. Abuse should be considered with:

- Any fracture without an adequate explanation.
- Any fracture in a non-ambulatory infant.
- Unusual fractures such as rib, metaphyseal and spinal (these fractures are rare in everyday life so have a high specificity for NAI).
- Multiple injuries over a period of time.
- Delayed presentation or an inconsistent clinical history.

NAI is a major cause of morbidity and mortality and the outcome is death in 2%, severe injury in 30%, re-injury in 10–30%, and the child is returned to their family 60% of the time. A vital part of the management of NAI involves keeping the child in a place of safety to await assessment by the child protection team.

The cases

Case 1

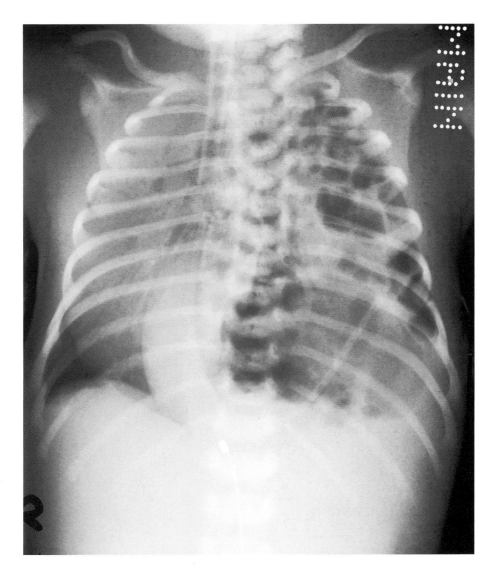

This term baby was admitted to the neonatal unit with respiratory distress.

1. What abnormalities are seen on the frontal chest radiograph?
2. What is the diagnosis?

ANSWERS

1. There are multiple lucencies in the left hemithorax, mediastinal shift to the right and there is little aeration of the right lung. The gastric bubble is not seen in the normal position and there is no bowel gas seen below the diaphragm. The tip of the nasogastric tube is in the left chest.
2. Left congenital diaphragmatic hernia, with multiple loops of bowel within the left hemithorax.

RADIOLOGY HOT LIST

- Initial radiographs may show an opaque hemithorax, as the bowel loops are fluid filled. As the baby swallows air, the characteristic gas-filled bowel loops appear in the thorax.
- Placement of a nasogastric tube verifies that the stomach is in the chest.
- The differential diagnosis of cystic intrathoracic lesions is congenital cystic adenomatoid malformation, where there is a normal abdominal bowel gas pattern and the NG tube is normally sited.
- Ultrasound can be helpful to confirm the presence of bowel loops within the chest and demonstrate the diaphragmatic defect. In doubtful cases, an upper GI contrast study can be performed.

CLINICAL HOT LIST

- Incidence 1 : 2500 live births, most diagnosed antenatally.
- 80% of herniations are left posterolateral (Bochdalek).
- Embryology: the pleuroperitoneal opening (foramen of Bochdalek) fails to close. Abdominal viscera herniate into the thorax, compromising pulmonary development.
- Morbidity depends on the degree of pulmonary hypoplasia and associated pulmonary hypertension: the presence of aerated lung on both sides is a good prognostic indicator.

FURTHER READING

Paterson A. 2005: Imaging evaluation of congenital lung abnormalities in infants and children. *Radiol Clin N Am;* 43: 303–23.
Smith NP, Jesudason EC, Fetherstone NC, Corbett NJ, Losty PD. 2005: Recent advances in congenital diaphragmatic hernia. *Arch Dis Child;* 90: 426–8.

Case 2

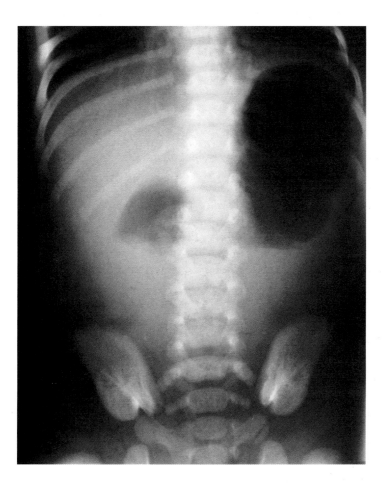

This baby was reviewed on the postnatal ward for poor feeding and bilious vomiting.

1. What abnormality is seen on the plain abdominal radiograph?
2. What is the most likely diagnosis?
3. With what condition is this associated?

ANSWERS

1. There is gas in the stomach and proximal duodenum but none elsewhere, giving the 'double-bubble' sign.
2. Duodenal atresia.
3. Down's syndrome.

RADIOLOGY HOT LIST

- Duodenal atresia represents a complete obstruction, with no gas seen beyond the duodenum. The abdominal X-ray is diagnostic and a contrast study is *not* required.
- If the abdominal radiograph suggests incomplete obstruction (with a small amount of gas in the distal bowel), a careful upper gastrointestinal (GI) contrast study should be performed to assess the site of obstruction, and exclude a malrotation/midgut volvulus, which is a surgical emergency.
- Other causes of neonatal duodenal obstruction include duodenal stenosis, duodenal web, annular pancreas, Ladd's bands and midgut volvulus, which all show gas in the distal bowel.

CLINICAL HOT LIST

- Incidence 1 : 1000 live births.
- The cause appears to be a failure in canalization of the fetal duodenum due to early developmental insult. There is a strong association with other abnormalities of the GI and biliary tracts, e.g. malrotation, oesophageal atresia and anal anomalies. Cardiac and renal abnormalities are sometimes seen.
- Up to 30% have Down's syndrome.
- Most atresias occur distal to the ampulla of Vater, presenting with bilious vomiting in the first few hours of life. An incomplete obstruction may present later.
- Antenatal diagnosis is possible; 40% will have maternal polyhydramnios.

FURTHER READING

Berrocal T, Torres I, Gutiérrez J, Prieto C, del Hoyo ML, Lamas M. 1999: Congenital anomalies of the upper gastrointestinal tract. *RadioGraphics;* 19: 855–72.

Naik-Mathuria B, Olutoyo OO. 2006: Foregut abnormalities. *Surg Clin N Am;* 86: 261–84.

Case 3

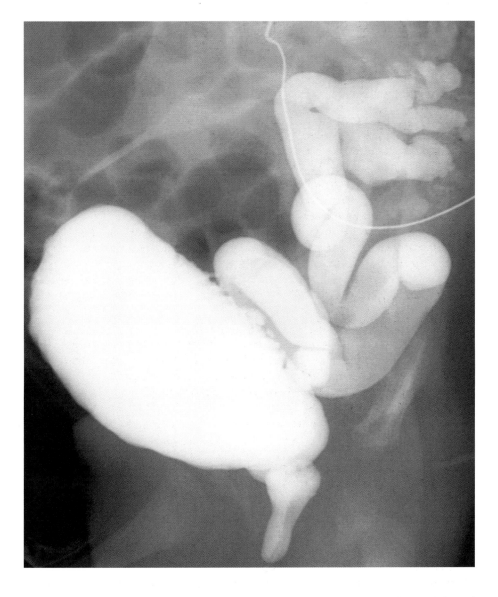

This 4-day-old boy is in renal failure. Antenatal ultrasound had shown bilateral hydronephrosis.

1. What investigation is this?
2. What does it show?
3. What is the diagnosis?

ANSWERS

1. A micturating cysto-urethrogram (MCUG).
2. There is an abrupt change in calibre of the urethra, with dilatation of the posterior urethra. The bladder wall is trabeculated. There is bilateral vesicoureteric reflux into dilated and tortuous ureters.
3. Posterior urethral valves.

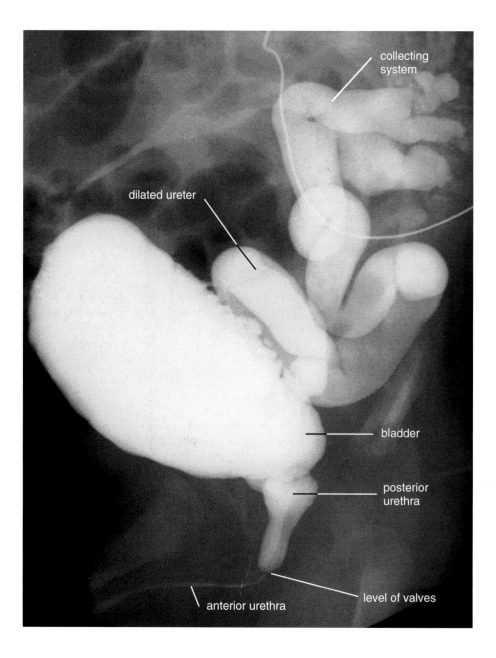

RADIOLOGY HOT LIST

- The diagnosis of posterior urethral valves is usually made on an MCUG. This will show dilatation of the posterior urethra, a transverse filling defect (valves) and reduction of the urethral calibre distal to the obstruction.
- The bladder may be large or small volume, with trabeculation of the bladder wall.
- Vesicoureteric reflux is common and associated with a worse prognosis. It occurs in approximately 50% and is bilateral in 15%.
- Antenatal ultrasound may suggest the diagnosis, showing dilatation of the ureters and pelvicalyceal systems and a thick-walled bladder. There may be oligohydraminios, which is associated with a worse prognosis.
- All children should receive antibiotic cover at the time of the MCUG. The investigation should not be performed in the presence of a urinary tract infection (UTI).

CLINICAL HOT LIST

- Valves are mucosal folds that close on voiding, leading to obstruction.
- It is rare, but remains the commonest obstructive uropathy in boys.
- There is a spectrum of severity from mild to severe. The condition is usually diagnosed antenatally or in the neonatal period, but milder forms may not present until later in childhood.
- Neonatal presentation may be with urinary retention, poor stream, infection or uraemia. Infants present more commonly with UTI.
- There is an association with renal dysplasia.
- Treatment is by surgical disruption of the valves. Prognosis depends on the duration and severity of obstruction prior to corrective surgery, and the presence of vesicoureteric reflux.
- If antenatally detected, obstruction may be relieved by percutaneous vesico-amniotic shunting.

FURTHER READING

Fernbach SK, Feinstein KA, Schmidt MB. 2000: Pediatric voiding cystourethrography: A pictorial guide. *RadioGraphics;* 20: 155–68.

Hutton KAR. 2004: Management of posterior urethral valves. *Curr Paediatr;* 14: 568–75.

Case 4

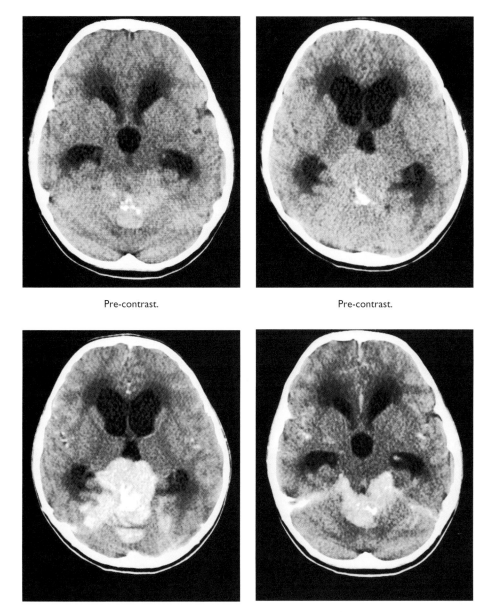

Pre-contrast.   Pre-contrast.

Post-contrast.   Post-contrast.

This 5-year-old boy was admitted with a 1-month history of headache and vomiting.

1. What does the CT scan show?
2. What is the most likely diagnosis?

ANSWERS

1. There is a midline solid mass in the posterior fossa, arising from the vermis and extending superiorly. It is partially calcified and shows marked enhancement after contrast. This is causing obstructive hydrocephalus (the periventricular low density indicates that this is acute).
2. Medulloblastoma.

RADIOLOGY HOT LIST

- Medulloblastoma is usually a well-defined posterior fossa mass arising from the cerebellar vermis in the midline. CT classically shows an intensely enhancing central solid mass.
- Encroachment on the IVth ventricle/aqueduct causes hydrocephalus in the majority.
- Subarachnoid metastatic spread results in deposits in the spinal cord, cauda equina and intracranial CSF spaces. These are best assessed with MRI. Metastases also occur to bone, lymph nodes and lung.
- The differential diagnosis of childhood posterior fossa masses includes ependymoma, cerebellar astrocytoma, haemangioblastoma and brainstem glioma.

CLINICAL HOT LIST

- Medulloblastoma accounts for 20% of childhood CNS tumours (peak incidence at 5 years of age).
- It commonly presents with signs of raised intracranial pressure secondary to obstructive hydrocephalus. Other features are progressive ataxia, diplopia, cranial nerve palsies, nuchal rigidity and head tilt, and deteriorating school performance.
- Prognostic features include tumour size, local extension and resectability, and presence of metastases.
- Surgical resection is required for diagnosis, to remove as much tumour as possible and to relieve hydrocephalus. Radiotherapy of the entire neural axis and chemotherapy are also employed.
- 70% of patients will be disease free at 5 years.
- Long-term problems include growth and endocrine abnormalities, behavioural and learning difficulties. Recurrence is not uncommon.

FURTHER READING

Koeller KK, Rushing EJ. 2003: From the Archives of the AFIP: Medulloblastoma: A comprehensive review with radiologic-pathologic correlation. *RadioGraphics;* 23: 1613–37.

Vloeberghs M. 2005: Decision making in paediatric brain tumours: A neurosurgical perspective. *Curr Paediatr;* 15: 406–11.

Case 5

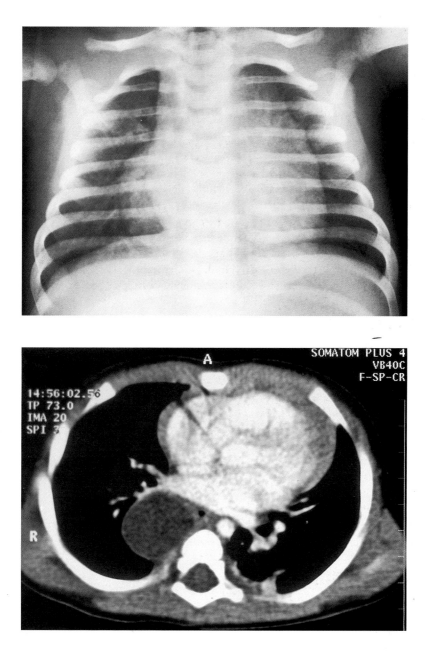

This 7-month-old girl suffers from recurrent chest infections. A chest x-ray and a CT chest scan have been performed.

1. What do they show?
2. What is the most likely diagnosis?

ANSWERS

1. The chest x-ray shows a sharply demarcated right paraspinal opacity. On CT there is a well-defined, thin-walled, fluid density lesion in the right side of the posterior mediastinum, which is intimately related to the oesophagus. The mass actually arises from the subcarinal region.
2. Foregut duplication (bronchogenic) cyst.

RADIOLOGY HOT LIST

- A cystic lesion at the level of the carina on CT/MRI is most commonly due to a bronchogenic cyst.
- Chest x-rays and CT scans show a well-defined cystic lesion typically lying in the middle or posterior mediastinum around the carina. Previous infection and haemorrhage can complicate the appearance, leading to a mixed density, solid appearance and air–fluid levels.
- MRI typically shows a homogeneous T2 high-signal mass. There is variable T1 intensity depending on the protein content of the cyst and the presence of blood products.

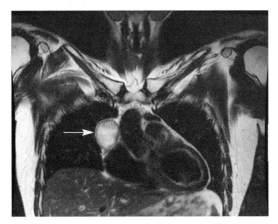

Coronal T2-weighted MRI shows a high signal bronchogenic cyst in the right mediastinum.

CLINICAL HOT LIST

- Bronchogenic cysts are rare congenital anomalies of ventral foregut development. They arise adjacent to the trachea and oesophagus, usually around the carina.
- Many are asymptomatic and detected as incidental findings on chest radiography.
- Symptoms may be due to compression of structures, including life-threatening airway compromise and stridor. Infection and haemorrhage may also occur.
- Treatment is by complete surgical excision.

FURTHER READING

Newman B. 2006: Congenital bronchopulmonary foregut malformations: concepts and controversies. *Pediatr Radiol;* 36: 773–91.

Takeda S, Miyoshi S, Minami M, et al. 2003: Clinical spectrum of mediastinal cysts. *Chest* 124: 125–32.

Case 6

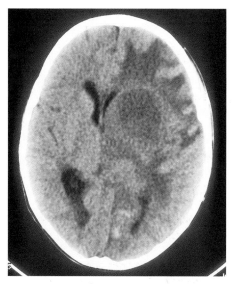

Pre-contrast.

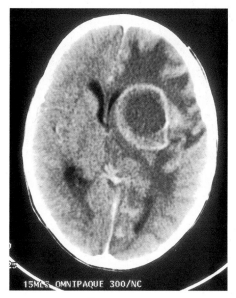

Post-contrast.

This febrile 8-year-old boy was admitted in status epilepticus. He had a 2-week history of sinusitis.

1. What abnormality is seen on the CT scan of the brain?
2. What is the diagnosis?

ANSWERS

1. There is a large ring-enhancing lesion surrounded by an area of low attenuation in the left frontal lobe. It is causing distortion of the anterior horn of the left lateral ventricle, and midline shift.
2. Left frontal cerebral abscess with surrounding cerebral oedema.

RADIOLOGY HOT LIST

- Large abscesses can be seen on non-contrast CT as an area of low attenuation with mass effect, occasionally with increased rim density due to the abscess wall. Gas within the lesion is diagnostic of gas-forming organisms.
- Contrast-enhanced CT increases the sensitivity and is more effective in demonstrating small multifocal abscesses, which may be missed on non-contrast scans.
- MRI is the most sensitive modality for detecting further abscesses.

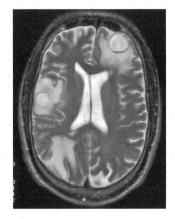

T2-weighted MRI showing brain abscesses.

CLINICAL HOT LIST

- Causes of intracerebral abscess:

  1. Contiguous suppurative focus: middle ear, sinuses, mastoid bone, odontogenic infection.
  2. Meningitis.
  3. Haematogenous spread: cyanotic congenital heart disease (R to L shunt), pulmonary suppuration, immunosuppression (may be multifocal).
  4. Trauma: compound skull fracture; penetrating wound to cranium, neurosurgery.

- Presentation is with headache, seizures, fever, altered level of consciousness. 70% have focal neurological signs. There may be signs of raised intracranial pressure.
- Cross-sectional imaging with contrast is the primary investigation. Lumbar puncture is dangerous and is not diagnostic.
- Management involves prolonged intravenous antibiotic therapy (including anaerobic cover) and neurosurgical consultation for drainage.

FURTHER READING

Xavier S. 2003: Brain abscesses in children. *Semin Paediatr Infect Dis;* 14: 108–14.

Case 7

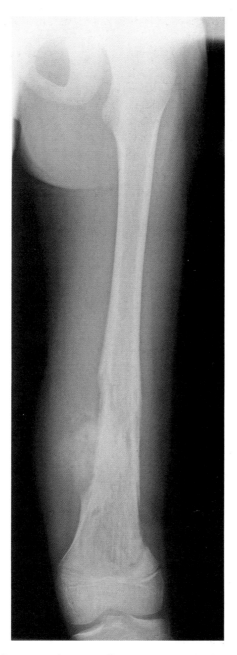

This 13-year-old girl presented to Accident & Emergency (A & E) with a 5-month history of pain in the left knee.

1. What does the plain film show?
2. What is the most likely diagnosis?

ANSWERS

1. There is an ill defined, partially calcified mass in the left distal femur, associated with an extensive permeative lucency of the femur, erosion of the bony cortex and soft tissue swelling.
2. Osteosarcoma of the distal femur.

RADIOLOGY HOT LIST

- Osteosarcomas are most commonly located in the long bone metaphyses. 70% occur around the knee.
- They may be sclerotic or lytic lesions. They are aggressive in appearance with poorly defined margins, cortical disruption and with a wide zone of transition between normal and abnormal bone.
- There is a periosteal reaction that is ill-defined and irregular, often with an associated ossifying soft tissue mass.
- MRI is required to evaluate bone marrow extension, vascular involvement, and the soft tissue component.
- A bone scan will demonstrate avid tracer uptake within the primary tumour and bony metastases, while chest CT is required to exclude pulmonary metastases (the most common site).

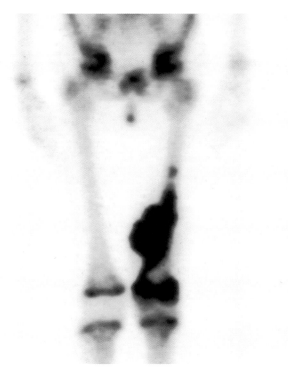

Bone scan shows the primary tumour in the distal left femur.

CLINICAL HOT LIST

- Osteosarcoma accounts for 60% of malignant bone tumours in childhood, in males more than in females, and with peak incidence in the second decade. They may be related to rapid growth in adolescence.
- The most common sites are in the metaphyses of long bones (in particular the distal femur, proximal tibia and humerus), pelvis and jaw.
- Predispositions and associations—chronic osteomyelitis, previous radiotherapy, retinoblastoma, bone dysplasia and chromosome 13 defect.
- Presentation is with bone pain and swelling, depending on the site. Systemic or other symptoms are rare, even when there are metastases.
- Treatment: surgical excision of primary lesion +/− lung metastases and chemotherapy (often before surgery to shrink the lesion and assist with limb sparing).
- The prognosis depends on tumour grade and site, extramedullary spread and metastases. A primary tumour in a distal extremity has a better prognosis than one in the axial skeleton. The 5-year survival rate is 65%.

FURTHER READING

Stacy GS, Mahal RS, Peabody TD. 2006: Staging of bone tumors: A review with illustrative examples. *AJR;* 186: 967–76.

Case 8

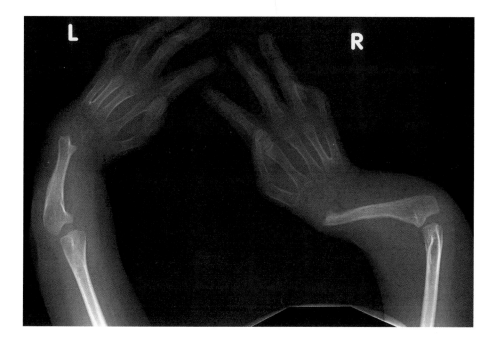

This child bruises easily.

1. What abnormality is seen on the X-ray of the forearms and hands?
2. What is the diagnosis?

ANSWERS

1. The radius is absent and the ulna is short on both sides. Both thumbs are hypoplastic.
2. Thrombocytopaenia–Absent Radius (TAR) syndrome.

RADIOLOGY HOT LIST

- Aplasia/hypoplasia of the radius is one of several limb reduction anomalies. Radial ray anomalies refer to the radius, first metacarpal, and thumb.

CLINICAL HOT LIST

- Inheritance is mostly sporadic. Thrombocytopaenia may remit in childhood.
- Absent radius is associated with:
  — Thromboctyopenia–Absent Radius (TAR) syndrome.
  — Fanconi's anaemia.
  — Holt-Oram syndrome.
  — **V**ertebral abnormalities, **A**nal atresia, **T**racheo**E**sophageal fistula, **R**enal or **L**imb abnormalities (VATER)/VACTERL.
  — Acrofacial dysostosis.
  — Thalidomide embryopathy.

FURTHER READING

Pharoah POD, Stevenson CJ, West CR. 2003: Thrombocytopenia – absent radius syndrome. *Arch Dis Childhood* 88: 295–8.

Case 9

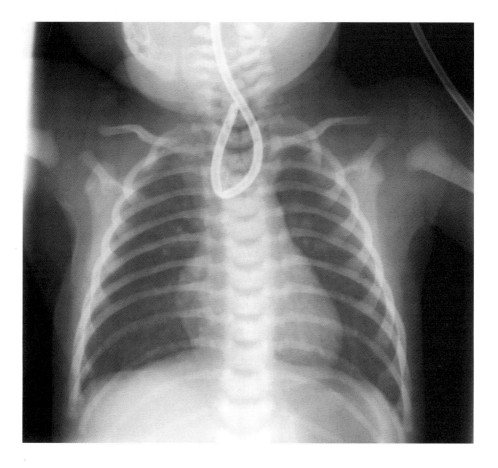

This 6-hour-old baby was admitted to the neonatal unit with choking and cyanosis during his first feed.

1. What abnormality is seen on the chest radiograph?
2. What is the diagnosis?

48

ANSWERS

1. The nasogastric tube is coiled in a dilated blind-ending proximal oesophagus. The gastric air bubble is present. The lungs are clear, with no evidence of aspiration.
2. Oesophageal atresia with a tracheo-oesophageal fistula.

RADIOLOGY HOT LIST

- The presence of the atresia is usually apparent on the plain chest x-ray, with a gas-filled proximal oesophageal pouch, usually ending at the junction of the upper one-third and lower two-thirds of the oesophagus. The presence of air in the stomach is indicative of a tracheo-oesophageal fistula.
- An oesophagram is usually performed to identify the site of fistulae, including the H-type fistula (2%) when there is a normally patent oesophagus.
- Remember the VATER/VACTERL association and look for associated anatomical anomalies.

CLINICAL HOT LIST

- Incidence is 1 : 3000, with associated malformations in up to 50% (VATER, VACTERL, CHARGE, trisomy 21, trisomy 18, DiGeorge syndrome).
- Antenatal clues include maternal polyhydramnios and an absent fetal stomach bubble.
- There are five anatomical variants (85% have oesophageal atresia with a distal tracheo-oesophageal fistula).
- Nurse prone and head up, with a Repolge tube on continuous suction in the oesophageal pouch to prevent aspiration.
- Surgical repair depends on oesophageal length: primary end-to-end anastomosis, or a staged repair to allow growth of segments, followed by gastric/colonic interposition.
- Survival will depend on the presence of other congenital abnormalities and birthweight. Oesophageal dysmotility may be a long-term sequela.

FURTHER READING

Berrocal T, Torres I, Gutierrez I et al. 1999: Congenital anomalies of the upper gastrointestinal tract. *RadioGraphics;* 19: 855–72.
Goyal A, Jones MO, Couriel JM, Losty PD. 2006: Oesophageal atresia and tracheo-oesophageal fistula. *Arch Dis Child;* 91: F381–8.

Case 10

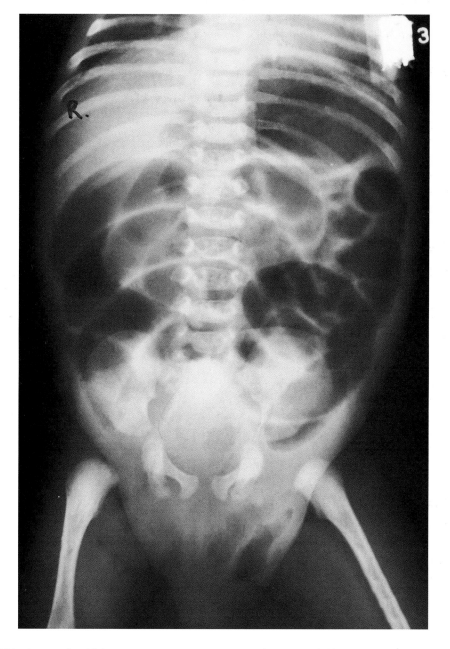

This 3-month-old boy was seen in A & E with inconsolable crying, abdominal distension and vomiting.

1. What abnormalities are seen on the abdominal radiograph?
2. What is the diagnosis?

ANSWERS

1. There are multiple loops of dilated gas-filled bowel. There is a gas shadow projected over the left hemiscrotum. No free air is seen.
2. Low bowel obstruction secondary to a left inguinal hernia.

RADIOLOGY HOT LIST

- It is difficult to distinguish between small and large bowel in neonates and infants. Obstruction is described as high or low, depending upon the anatomical location and number of visible bowel loops.
- If the distended bowel loops are fluid filled, the abdomen may have a 'gasless' appearance.
- Always look for intrascrotal air as incarcerated inguinal hernias are the most common cause of low bowel obstruction in infants younger than 6 months (excluding the neonatal period).
- Look for free intraperitoneal air secondary to perforation.

CLINICAL HOT LIST

- Inguinal hernias are common in infancy. The incidence is >10 : 1000 live births, and they occur more in males than females, more on the left side than the right, and 10% are bilateral.
- They are caused by failure of closure of the processus vaginalis, resulting in an indirect hernia (through the inguinal canal). Direct inguinal hernias are very rare in childhood.
- Associations include congenital genitourinary abnormality, prematurity, low birthweight, abdominal wall defect and anything that increases intra-abdominal pressure, e.g. ascites.
- All inguinal hernias will require surgery. If irreducible there is a risk of strangulation (bowel ischaemia), which requires immediate surgical intervention.
- Adhesions are the most common cause of obstruction in babies who have had previous neonatal surgery.
- Other causes of low GI obstruction in infants include intussusception, short segment Hirschprung's disease, ileal or colonic stenoses (strictures following necrotizing enterocolitis), or extrinsic masses (duplication cysts and appendix abscess).

FURTHER READING

Davenport M. 1996: ABC of general paediatric surgery. Inguinal hernia, hydrocele and the undescended testis. *BMJ;* 312: 564–71.

Case 11

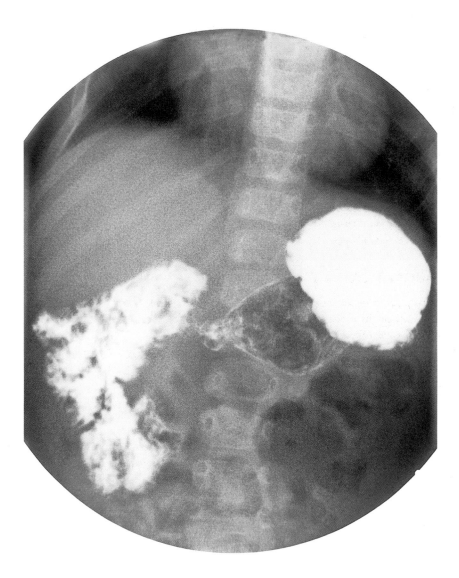

A 2-day-old boy is reviewed on the postnatal ward. Breast-feeding is well established and he has passed a small amount of meconium on day 1. There is now a 6-hour history of bile-stained vomiting.

1. What is this study?
2. What abnormality is demonstrated?
3. What is the diagnosis?

ANSWERS

1. An upper gastrointestinal contrast study.
2. The duodenum, duodeno-jejunal (DJ) flexure and proximal small bowel loops are abnormally sited, lying to the right of the midline.
3. Malrotation.

RADIOLOGY HOT LIST

- An upper GI contrast study is the definitive investigation to identify the presence and location of an obstruction.
- The position of the duodeno-jejunal flexure is critical in the diagnosis of malrotation. It should lie to the left of the midline, at the level of the pylorus. The proximal jejunal loops should be left sided (see page 12).
- Midgut volvulus may occur, resulting in the small bowel having a 'corkscrew' appearance, as it twists around the superior mesenteric artery.

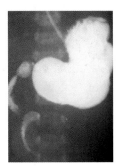

A midgut volvulus, with a typical cockscrew appearance.

- Reversal of the position of the superior mesenteric artery and vein on ultrasound may suggest malrotation, but is not definitive.

CLINICAL HOT LIST

- Malrotation and midgut volvulus are neonatal surgical emergencies, and need to be excluded in neonatal bilious vomiting. 60–80% of cases present in the first month of life.
- Malrotation is an abnormality of small bowel rotation and fixation. The normal small bowel mesentery should be fixed from the DJ flexure in the left upper quadrant to the caecum in the right iliac fossa. In malrotation the mesentery is abnormally sited and narrow, allowing the small bowel to twist around a narrow pedicle (a volvulus).
- The superior mesenteric artery is contained in the twisted mesentery, leading to small bowel ischaemia and potential infarction.
- Obstruction may be intermittent, and the diagnosis should be considered in older children with similar symptoms.

FURTHER READING

Applegate KE, Anderson JM, Klatte EC. 2006: Intestinal malrotation in children: A problem-solving approach to the upper gastrointestinal series. *RadioGraphics;* 2006; 26: 1485–1500.

Williams H. 2007: Green for Danger! Intestinal malrotation and volvulus. *Arch Dis Child;* 92: ep87–91.

Case 12

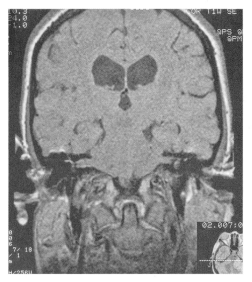

(a) Pre-contrast.

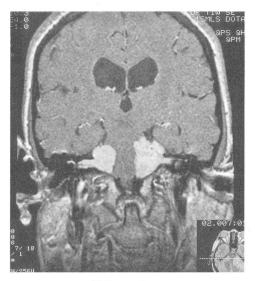

(b) Post-contrast.

This 18-year-old female, with an inherited disorder, had a progressive onset of bilateral sensorineural deafness. An MRI brain scan was obtained.

1. What abnormalities are seen on the coronal T1-weighted images pre- and post-enhancement?
2. What is the diagnosis?
3. What is the underlying condition?

ANSWERS

1. There are bilateral isointense masses (on T1 weighting) at the cerebello-pontine angles that show intense enhancement with gadolinium. The masses extend into and expand the internal auditory canals bilaterally. The pons is compressed.
2. Bilateral acoustic neuromas.
3. Neurofibromatosis type 2.

RADIOLOGY HOT LIST

- Acoustic neuromas are schwannomas that arise from the vestibular (VIII) nerve. They may arise within, or at the opening of the internal auditory canal, and classically expand and erode the internal acoustic meatus.
- There may be obliteration of the ipsilateral cerebellopontine (CP) angle cistern, compression of the pons and distortion of the IVth ventricle with associated hydrocephalus.
- The mass is usually non-calcified, and shows intense enhancement on both CT and MRI.
- Acoustic neuromas account for 80% of CP angle tumours. The main differential diagnosis is a meningioma.

CLINICAL HOT LIST

- Bilateral acoustic neuromas allow a presumptive diagnosis of neurofibromatosis type 2 (NF2).
- NF2 is an autosomal dominant, multisystem, genetic disorder, distinct from NF1. The gene location is on chromosome 22q. The incidence 1 : 37,000; 50% are new mutations.
- Clinical features of acoustic neuromas include slowly progressive deafness, imbalance, tinnitus, cerebellar ataxia, features of raised intracranial pressure and other cranial nerve palsies.
- NF2 is associated with few skin changes (unlike NF1). These include < 5 café-au-lait spots and subcutaneous schwannomas (neurofibromas in NF1). Meningiomas, ependymomas and cataracts can also occur.

FURTHER READING

Patronas NJ, Courcoutsakis N, Bromley CM et al. 2001: Intramedullary and spinal canal tumors in patients with neurofibromatosis 2: MR imaging findings and correlation with genotype. *Radiology*; 2001; 218: 434.

Case 13

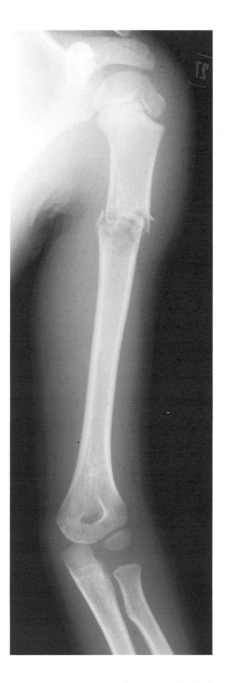

This 4-year-old boy presented to A & E with pain in the left upper arm following a relatively trivial fall.

1. What does the X-ray show?
2. What is the most likely diagnosis?

ANSWERS

1. There is a fracture through the proximal humerus at the site of a well-defined lytic lesion.
2. A pathological fracture through a simple bone cyst.

RADIOLOGY HOT LIST

- Simple bone cysts are characteristically well-defined, expanded lytic lesions, with a thin but intact bony cortex.
- They are commonly found in the proximal humerus and proximal femur, and are usually asymptomatic unless a pathological fracture occurs. They may be incidental findings on plain radiographs, and usually involute with time.
- Fibrous dysplasia can mimic these appearances radiologically.
- Aneurysmal bone cysts are larger expansile lesions of bone, containing blood-filled thin-walled cavities. They do not cross the epiphyseal plate, and often present with pain or pathological fracture.

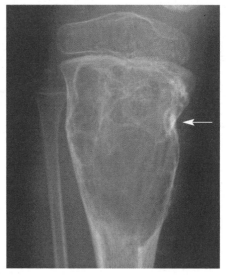

An aneurysmal bone cyst of the proximal tibia, with a subtle linear sclerotic line indicating a pathological fracture.

CLINICAL HOT LIST

- Simple bone cysts originate at the epiphyseal plate in long bones and grow into the shaft of the bone, changing position with skeletal maturity. They are rarely seen after the age of 30.
- 50% will present with a pathological fracture. Occasionally growth arrest can be seen.
- If symptomatic they may require curettage and bone packing, or intra-lesional steroid injection.

FURTHER READING

Miller SL, Hoffer FA. 2001: Malignant and benign bone tumors. *Radiol Clin N Am;* 39: 673–99.

Case 14

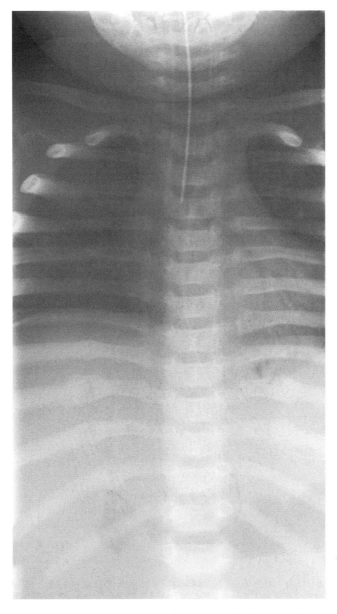

This 6-month-old baby was admitted having collapsed at home. There was a history of a visit to another casualty department with a similar episode. This is a post-intubation film.

1. What abnormality is seen on the chest x-ray?
2. What is the significance?
3. What further imaging should be performed?

58

ANSWERS

1. There are bilateral healing fractures of the posterior ribs with associated callus formation.
2. These features are highly suggestive of non-accidental injury (NAI).
3. A dedicated skeletal survey and CT of the brain will be required.

RADIOLOGY HOT LIST

- Rib fractures are rare in childhood, as the compressive forces required are considerable. Unless there is a history of significant trauma (e.g. a road traffic accident), rib fractures in children under the age of 3 years are almost always due to NAI.
- Rib fractures result from severe compressive forces to the rib cage or as a result of a direct blow to the chest. Rib fractures are therefore regarded as 'high specificity' fractures.
- Rib fractures may not be visible immediately. Since they heal with callus formation, delayed films at 10 days may show occult fractures. Always consider delayed films if there is a high index of suspicion with a normal chest x-ray.
- A bone scan may be positive within hours of injury. It may be useful to confirm the presence of subtle rib fractures and may highlight other injuries.
- Metaphyseal fractures are also highly suggestive of NAI.

CLINICAL HOT LIST

- The true incidence of NAI is unknown. It is likely that there is significant underreporting of child abuse, and it remains a major cause of morbidity and mortality.
- There is often inadequate explanation for injuries, inconsistencies in the history and delayed presentation. There may be multiple injuries with presentation to different hospitals.
- Physical abuse may involve the brain and/or the skeletal system.
- Infants may present with cerebral injury as a consequence of shaking +/– impact. Presentations include collapse, apnoeas, seizures, acute life-threatening events and death.
- Older children more commonly present with fractures. Fractures are also common in infants, and may be associated with brain injury.
- After dealing with the injuries, a full skeletal survey and a CT of the brain should be performed.
- The child should be kept in a place of safety to await assessment by the child protection team.

FURTHER READING

Royal College of Radiologists and Royal College of Paediatrics and Child Health. 2008: Standards for Radiological Investigations of Suspected Non-accidental Injury.
Speight N. 2006: Child abuse. *Curr Paed;* 16: 100–5.
Williams RL, Connolly PT. 2004: In children undergoing chest radiography, what is the specificity of rib fractures for non-accidental injury? *Arch Dis Child;* 89: 490–2.

Case 15

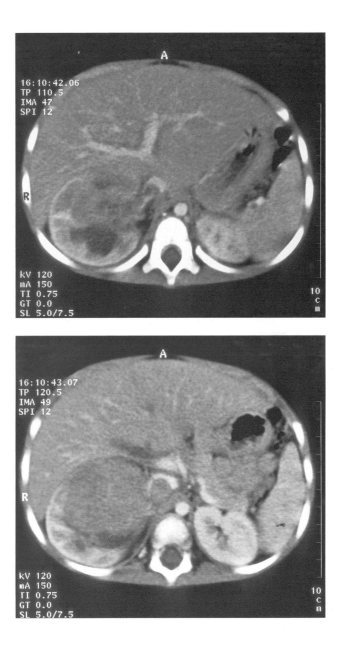

The parents of this 3-year-old boy noticed an abdominal mass when they were giving him a bath.

1. What abnormalities are seen on this contrast-enhanced CT scan of the abdomen?
2. What is the likely diagnosis?
3. What are the associated risk factors for this condition?

ANSWERS

1. There is a large, poorly enhancing, mixed-attenuation mass arising from the right kidney. No calcification is seen. There is a filling defect within the right renal vein and inferior vena cava (IVC) representing tumour invasion. The other blood vessels are displaced by the mass. The liver and left kidney appear normal on these images.

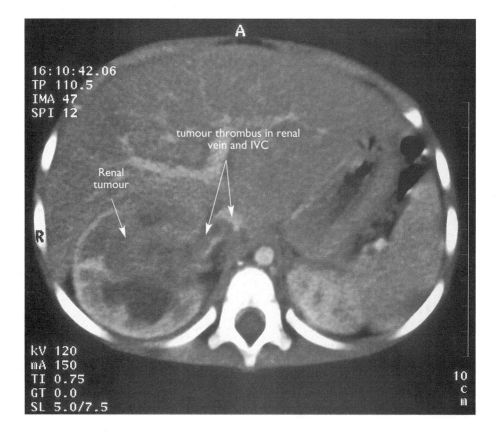

2. Wilms tumour.
3. Aniridia, genitourinary abnormalities, Denys–Drash syndrome, WAGR syndrome, Beckwith–Wiedemann syndrome, hemihypertrophy, chromosome 11 point deletion.

RADIOLOGY HOT LIST

- Wilms tumours are bilateral in 5%.
- The tumour usually has well-defined margins and classically displaces adjacent vessels, as opposed to encasing them (as with neuroblastoma).

- 5% have tumour thrombus in the renal vein and IVC.
- The plain abdominal radiograph may show enlargement of the renal outline and displacement of the adjacent bowel gas. Calcification is rare (10%).
- Pulmonary metastases are present in 10% at diagnosis.

CLINICAL HOT LIST

- Incidence 1 : 100,000 live births, M = F, most under 7 years (peak 3 years).
- Presentation is usually in a well child with a non-tender abdominal mass. 25% have haematuria, 5% hypertension.
- The disease staging is as follows:

Stage	Characteristics	10-year survival
I	One kidney, capsule intact, complete excision	98%
II	Extension beyond capsule, complete excision	96%
III	Residual tumour within abdomen	95%
IV	Haematogenous spread, e.g. lung, bone, liver	90%
V	Bilateral renal tumours	70%

- Management comprises surgery, chemotherapy and radiotherapy depending on staging.
- Long-term follow up is needed, to screen for recurrence and a second malignancy.

FURTHER READING

Lowe LH, Isuani BH, Heller RH et al. 2000: Pediatric renal masses: Wilms tumor and beyond. *RadioGraphics;* 20: 1585–1603.

Pritchard-Jones K. 2002: Controversies and advances in the management of Wilms tumour. *Arch Dis Child;* 87: 241–4.

Case 16

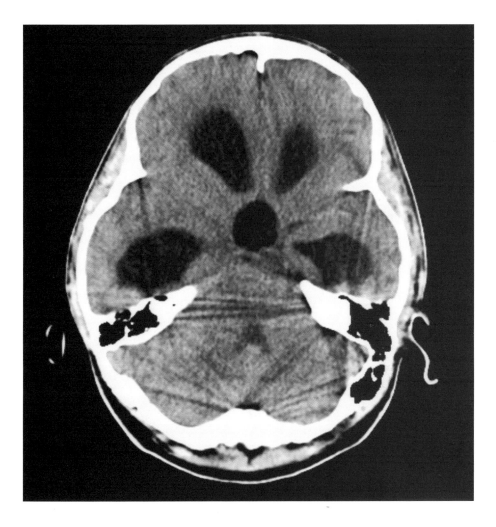

This 8-year-old boy has a large head and mild developmental delay.

1. Describe the abnormalities on the CT scan.
2. What is the condition?
3. What is the most likely cause?

ANSWERS

1. There is marked dilatation of the lateral and third ventricles with a normal-sized fourth ventricle. There is no mass lesion.
2. Non-communicating hydrocephalus.
3. Congenital aqueduct stenosis.

RADIOLOGY HOT LIST

- Dilatation of the lateral (note the dilated temporal horns) and third ventricles with a normal-sized fourth ventricle indicates that the level of obstruction is at the aqueduct of Sylvius.
- Congenital aqueduct stenosis is the commonest cause of congenital hydrocephalus.
- There is no periventricular low density (which would indicate acute hydrocephalus), implying a longstanding abnormality.

CLINICAL HOT LIST

- Hydrocephalus is due to an imbalance of CSF production and reabsorption.
- Obstructive hydrocephalus is due to obstruction of the normal CSF flow and/or reabsorption. Overproduction of CSF (secondary to choroid plexus papilloma) is rare.

Type of obstructive hydrocephalus	Pathophysiology	Example
Communicating	Extraventricular blockage occurs beyond the fourth ventricle within the subarachnoid pathways and arachnoid granulations. All ventricles are dilated	Post-meningitis, post-haemorrhage
Non-communicating	Ventricular blockage with dilatation of ventricles proximal to obstruction	Arnold–Chiari II malformation, Dandy–Walker malformation, vein of Galen aneurysm, tumour

- The clinical presentation will vary with age and aetiology. Chronic presentation may include increasing head circumference, developmental delay and behavioural changes. An acute decompensation may present with signs of raised intracranial pressure, seizures and acute squint.
- Management involves neurosurgery and ventricular shunting.

FURTHER READING

Dineen RA, Jaspan T. 2006: Neuroimaging in children. *Curr Paed;* 16: 348–59.

Case 17

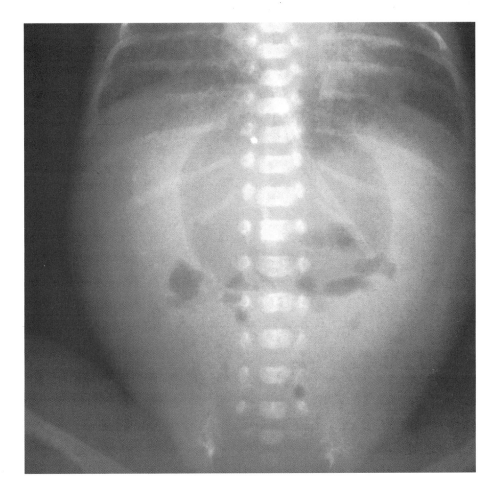

This 5-day-old neonate, born at 34 weeks' gestation and ventilated for surfactant deficiency disease has abdominal distension, metabolic acidosis and cardiovascular collapse.

1. What does the abdominal radiograph show?
2. What is the diagnosis?

ANSWERS

1. There is a large lucency projected over the upper abdomen due to free intraperitoneal air.
2. Acute GI perforation (usually secondary to necrotizing enterocolitis).

RADIOLOGY HOT LIST

- Free intraperitoneal air may not lie under the diaphragm when the patient is supine. It will collect in the least dependent area (adjacent to the anterior abdominal wall), resulting in a central rounded lucency ('football sign'). This may be quite subtle.
- Air may outline the falciform ligament, which appears as a linear density in the midline or right upper quadrant. This is more common than the football sign.

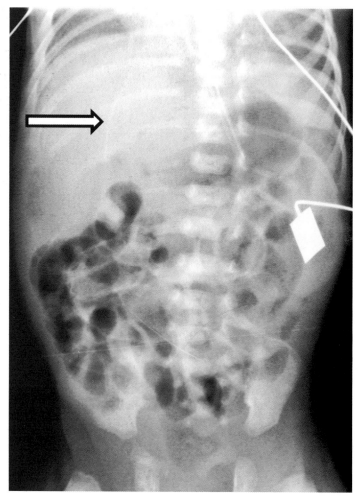

The falciform ligament with free air on either side.

- The bowel wall may be seen clearly as a thin white line if there is air on both sides of it (Rigler's sign).
- A horizontal beam 'shoot-through' film of the supine baby will show free air adjacent to the anterior abdominal wall, or a lateral decubitus film with the infant lying left side down will show free air surrounding the liver edge in equivocal cases.
- Remember that the upper abdomen is a key review area on a CXR, and the signs of free air may be very subtle.

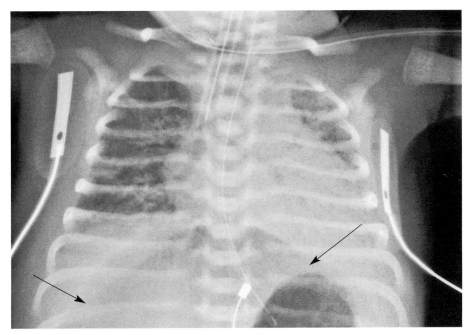

Free air below the diaphragm.

CLINICAL HOT LIST

- Major causes of neonatal perforation include necrotizing enterocolitis, Hirschsprung's disease, bowel atresia, imperforate anus and meconium ileus. Idiopathic and iatrogenic (oxygen connected to nasogastric tube) cases have been reported.
- Clinical features may be subtle, leading to a delay in recognition. The mortality rate is 17–60%.
- Management includes resuscitation and prompt surgical intervention.

FURTHER READING

Farrugia MK, Morgan AS, McHugh K, Kiely EM. 2003: Neonatal gastrointestinal perforation. *Arch Dis Child Fetal Neonatal Ed;* 88: 75.

Case 18

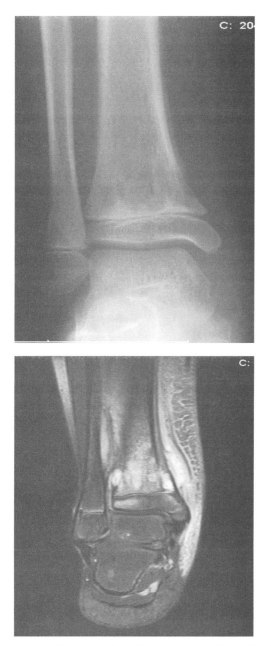

A 9-year-old boy was brought to the A & E department. He had a 10-day history of a painful right ankle. Clinically he was febrile and the right ankle was tender and erythematous. An X-ray and an MRI scan of the right ankle have been performed.

1. What does the X-ray show?
2. What does the T2-weighted MRI scan show?
3. What is the likely diagnosis?

ANSWERS

1. There is ill-defined lucency in the medial aspect of the right tibial metaphysis. This is associated with a periosteal reaction along the distal tibia, and adjacent soft tissue swelling.
2. There is high signal in the distal tibia, indicative of bone marrow oedema. There is elevation of the periosteum, with a high signal subperiosteal collection visible. There is high signal in the subcutaneous tissues, indicating oedema and a focal collection.
3. Acute osteomyelitis of the right ankle.

RADIOLOGY HOT LIST

- A plain film is usually the first-line investigation, although X-rays are often normal in acute osteomyelitis or show only subtle change. It may take up to 10 days before plain film changes are seen. In neonates X-ray changes may occur much earlier.
- Ultrasound is useful, particularly in the neonate and young child, to exclude associated septic arthritis, and may identify subperiosteal or soft tissue collections.
- MRI is the imaging modality of choice for confirming the diagnosis. It may show collections amenable to drainage in the bone marrow, subperiosteum or soft tissues. MRI cannot cover the entire skeleton, and may require sedation or general anaesthesia.
- A technetium bone scan is a useful tool if MRI is unavailable, and is usually positive early in the disease process, before plain film changes occur. The bone scan also has a role in the neonate with osetomyelitis, where multifocal disease is common. The disadvantage of a bone scan is the lack of anatomical information, and the radiation dose.

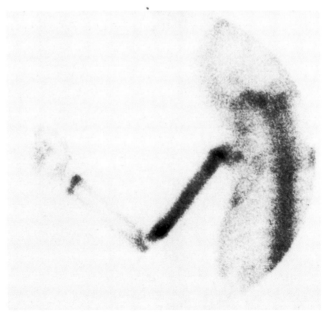

Bone scan showing avid tracer uptake in the right humerus due to osteomyelitis.

CLINICAL HOT LIST

- Acute osteomyelitis usually occurs secondary to haematogenous spread in children, but can occur due to contiguous spread, penetrating injury or surgery. Subacute and chronic osteomyelitis usually occurs as a consequence of inadequate treatment, low virulence organisms or underlying immunodeficiency:

Population	Organism
Infant	*Staphylococcus aureus*, group B *Streptococcus*, Gram–negative bacteria *Neisseria gonorrhoea*
Child	*S. aureus* (70%), *Streptococcus*, *N. meningitides*, *Haemophilus* (now rare)
Sickle cell disease	*Salmonella*

- Osteomyelitis usually presents with sudden onset of local bone pain, swelling, erythema, and immobility. Long bones are most commonly affected. The child is systemically unwell with fever and malaise. Blood cultures are positive in 60%.
- 50% of cases occur in preschool-aged children.
- Parenteral bacteriocidal antibiotics are needed initially. Antibiotic therapy for 6 weeks is usually required to eradicate infection. Early orthopaedic involvement is important as surgical drainage of bony or joint collections may be required, and may aid a microbiological diagnosis.

FURTHER READING

Foster K. 2004: The limping child. *Imaging;* 16: 153–60.
Vazquez M. 2002: Osteomyelitis in children. *Curr Opin Pediatr;* 14: 112–15.

Case 19

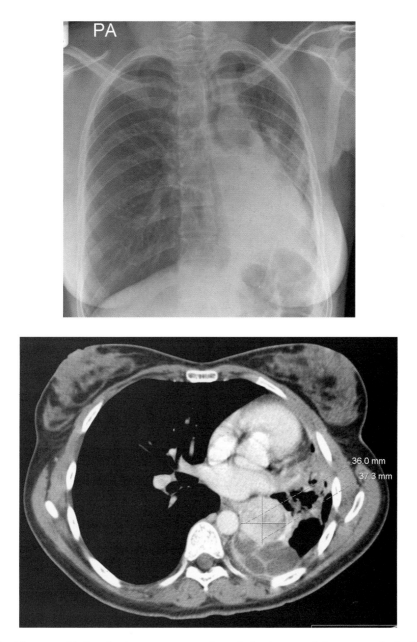

This 15-year-old female has recurrent chest infections and has recently had an episode of haemoptysis. A CXR and CT scan of the chest have been performed.

1. What does the CXR show?
2. What does the CT scan show?
3. What is the differential diagnosis?

ANSWERS

1. The CXR shows volume loss in the left hemithorax, with mediastinal shift to the left and elevation and loss of clarity of the left hemidiaphragm. There is opacification in the left mid and lower zones. The appearances are consistent with left lower lobe collapse/consolidation.
2. The CT scan shows a large avidly enhancing mass at the left hilum, which is obstructing the left lower lobe bronchus and causing collapse/consolidation of the left lower lobe (which contains dilated fluid-filled bronchi). There is mediastinal shift to the left.
3. This mass is a carcinoid tumour, but other causes of central obstructing masses would include a primary lung tumour, hilar lymphadenopathy (TB, lymphoma, metastatic adenopathy), and foregut duplication cysts.

RADIOLOGY HOT LIST

● Lobar collapse may be due to proximal airway obstruction:

Cause of proximal airway obstruction	Example
Intraluminal	Sputum plug, inhaled foreign body
Bronchial wall	Tumour
Extra-bronchial	Lymphadenopathy (TB, lymphoma), extrinsic mass (bronchogenic cyst)

● 80% of bronchial carcinoid tumours arise in lobar or main segmental bronchi. Tumour growth into the lumen may cause bronchial obstruction, recurrent segmental pneumonia, bronchiectasis, haemoptysis, and eventually collapse of the lung peripheral to the tumour.

CLINICAL HOT LIST

● Carcinoid tumours are rare neuroendocrine tumours derived from primitive stem cells of the embryonic gut. Potential sites include the lung, trachea, bronchus, thymus, GI tract, ovary and testis. The commonest site is the appendix (usually an incidental finding).
● Symptoms will vary with size, location, and metastatic spread and with the production of an array of bioactive substances, such as serotonin, catecholamines, histamine, 5-hydroxytryptamine and many others. These produce intermittent symptoms of flushing, tachycardia, altered blood pressure, pain, diarrhoea and wheeze.
● Surgical excision is the main treatment; chemotherapy is rarely required for metastatic disease.

FURTHER READING

Spunt SL, Pratt CB, Rao BN et al. 2000: Childhood carcinoid tumors: The St Jude Children's Research Hospital experience. *J Pediatr Surg;* 35: 1282–6.

Case 20

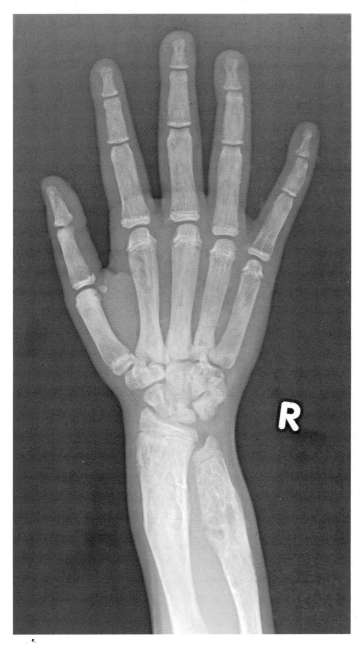

This 6-year-old girl has hyperpigmented areas of skin and precocious puberty.

1. What does the plain X-ray of the hand and wrist show?
2. What is the diagnosis?
3. What is the underlying condition?

ANSWERS

1. There are modelling defects of the bones with well-defined, expansile lytic lesions in the distal radius and ulna, and less marked changes in the metacarpals and phalanges. There are no associated soft tissue masses or periosteal reaction.
2. Polyostotic fibrous dysplasia.
3. McCune–Albright syndrome.

RADIOLOGY HOT LIST

- Benign bony lesions are classically well defined (a 'narrow zone of transition'). They typically expand the bone (implying slow growth) rather than destroy it. There should be no associated aggressive periosteal reaction or soft tissue mass present.
- The proximal femur is a typical location for fibrous dysplasia, where it may cause modelling deformities, leading to a 'shepherd's crook' appearance. The lesion may have an internal ground-glass (hazy) appearance.

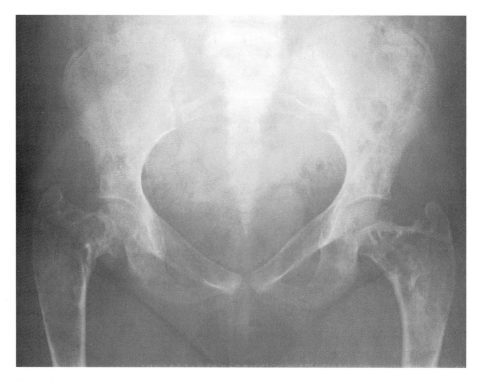

Similar changes in the pelvis and proximal femora resulting in bilateral coxa vara.

- Other bones affected by fibrous dysplasia include the skull and facial bones (typically sclerotic lesions), ribs and pelvis.

CLINICAL HOT LIST

- McCune–Albright syndrome is a triad of polyostotic fibrous dysplasia, skin pigmentation and autonomous endocrine hyperfunction—commonly precocious puberty. Other endocrine abnormalities include Cushings, hyperthyroidism, and gigantism/acromegaly.
- The skin lesions are 'coast of Maine' café-au-lait spots, seen on the back, trunk, shoulders and buttocks.
- Fibrous dysplasia is a developmental anomaly of the mesenchymal precursor of bone, causing areas of immature collagen matrix with small irregular bony trabeculae within the medullary cavity. It can affect long bones, spine or skull.
- The bone lesions may be asymptomatic, cause pain and limp, or may be disfiguring and impinge on vision or hearing.

FURTHER READING

Zacharin M. 2007: The spectrum of McCune–Albright syndrome. *Paediatr Endocrinol Rev;* 4(Suppl 4): 412–18.

Case 21

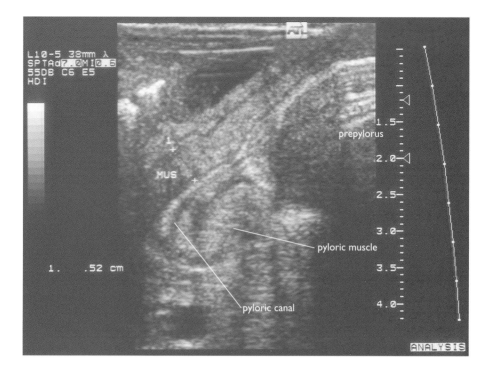

This 6 week old boy was admitted with vomiting after feeds and weight loss. On examination, he was hungry and wasted. Visible peristalsis was observed.

1. What examination has been performed?
2. What is the most likely diagnosis?

ANSWERS

1. Abdominal ultrasound to assess the pylorus.
2. Hypertrophic pyloric stenosis.

RADIOLOGY HOT LIST

- Ultrasound is the investigation of choice, though the diagnosis is often made clinically.
- The findings are of an enlarged and elongated pylorus, classically >17mm in longitudinal section, or >15mm in transverse section. The pyloric muscle thickness is >3mm. Borderline measurements are seen early in the disease and with premature infants.
- The area should be scanned continuously during a feed to demonstrate lack of opening of the pyloric canal with exaggerated peristalsis. This is the most sensitive imaging finding for this condition.
- A barium meal may show shouldering of the antrum with elongation and narrowing of the pyloric canal ('string sign').

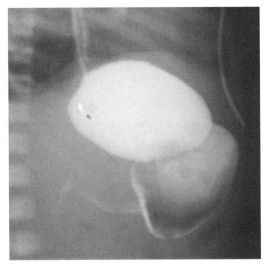

CLINICAL HOT LIST

- The condition is due to idiopathic hypertrophy of the circular muscle of the pylorus.
- It classically affects firstborn males at 2–8 weeks of life.
- Presentation is with non-bilious projectile vomiting, inadequate weight gain and a hungry baby.
- Clinical examination of the abdomen during feeding may demonstrate visible peristalsis, and the enlarged pylorus may be felt as a palpable 'olive-shaped' mass.
- Surgical pyloromyotomy is curative. Medical management with IV atropine is controversial.

FURTHER READING

Hernanz-Schulman M. Infantile hypertrophic pyloric stenosis. *Radiology*. May 2003; 227(2): 319-31.

Case 22

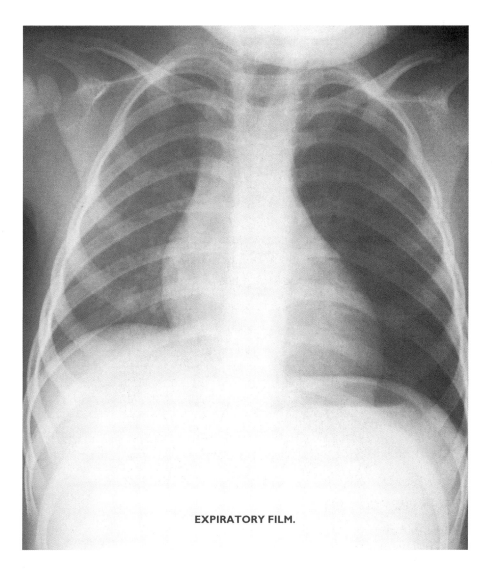

EXPIRATORY FILM.

This 2-year-old boy was seen in A & E with sudden onset of coughing and acute respiratory distress.

1. What does the chest radiograph show?
2. What is the most likely diagnosis?

ANSWERS

1. The left lung is of greater volume and is hyperlucent compared to the right. As the film is deliberately taken in expiration, this implies air trapping on the left. The normal right lung is smaller because it is an expiratory film. (Don't get caught out—it can be difficult to tell which side is abnormal.)
2. Inhaled foreign body in the left main bronchus (a peanut).

RADIOLOGY HOT LIST

- The normal cross-sectional diameter of the airway increases in inspiration and decreases in expiration. Foreign bodies can cause three radiological appearances according to their size:

Small	Normal CXR, no obstruction to air flow
Intermediate	Hyperinflation due to air trapping. Occlusion occurs in expiration only, due to normal decrease in bronchial diameter around the foreign body
Large	Distal consolidation and atelectasis due to complete obstruction of airway

- Depending upon the size of the foreign body, the site of impaction and the presence/absence of bronchospasm, there may be a variety of radiographic abnormalities including air trapping, atelectasis, consolidation, oligaemia, or a mixture of these findings.
- Confirmation of the diagnosis may be difficult. Children unable to cooperate with expiratory films can be assessed for air trapping with screening or decubitus views (lying on the suspect side, which would normally reduce in volume but remains hyperinflated due to the presence of a foreign body).
- Pneumomediastinum and pneumothorax are potential complications. Bronchiectasis may result from a missed foreign body.
- 90% of foreign bodies are not radio-opaque (usually organic material) and are thus not usually seen on the CXR.

CLINICAL HOT LIST

- This usually occurs in infants and children under the age of 4 years (M > F).
- They commonly present with sudden choking, cough and wheeze, which may subsequently settle. Delayed presentation occurs in up to 30%.
- The treatment of choice is bronchoscopic removal of the foreign body.

FURTHER READING

Franquet T, Giménez A, Rosón N et al. 2000: Aspiration diseases: findings, pitfalls, and differential diagnosis. *RadioGraphics;* 20: 673–85.
Williams H. 2005: Inhaled foreign bodies. *Arch Dis Child Ed Pract;* 90: ep31–33.

Case 23

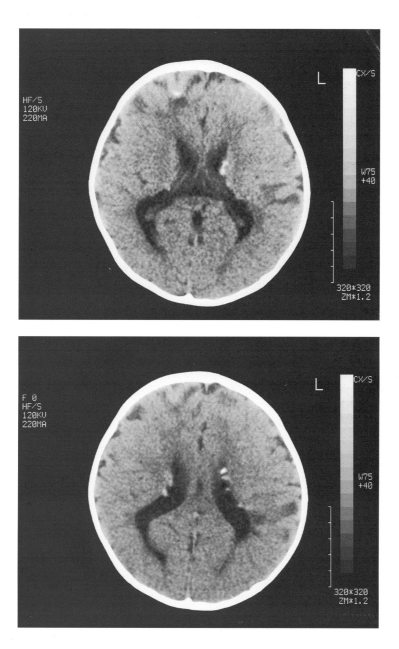

A 3-month-old girl presented with a history of frequent seizures. Investigations included a CT scan of the brain.

1. What abnormalities are present on the non-enhanced scan?
2. What is the diagnosis?

ANSWERS

1. There are multiple calcified subependymal nodules with a 'candle drippings' appearance along the lining of the lateral ventricles. There are several areas of low attenuation in the cerebral cortex that represent cortical tubers, one of which is calcified.
2. Tuberous sclerosis.

RADIOLOGY HOT LIST

- The typical findings in tuberous sclerosis are subependymal hamartomas protruding into the lateral ventricles. These calcify with increasing age.
- There may be cortical or subcortical hamartomas (tubers), which are typically non-calcified. The lesions are best demonstrated on MRI.

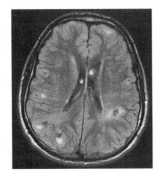

MRI brain showing multiple subcortical and subependymal hamartomas.

- 5–15% will develop a giant cell astrocytoma at the foramen of Munro, usually causing hydrocephalus.
- Other causes of intracerebral calcification at this age include intrauterine cytomegalovirus and toxoplasmosis infection. These will not show the typical subependymal location.

CLINICAL HOT LIST

- Tuberous sclerosis is an autosomal dominant condition. 50% result from spontaneous mutation.
- Cardinal features include multiple facial angiofibromas (adenoma sebaceum), subungual fibromas, retinal hamartomas and cortical tubers.
- Clinical expression is very variable—from minor skin changes seen in adult life to intractable epilepsy in infancy.
- Cutaneous features include 'ash leaf' white macules, which fluoresce under Woods light, and shagreen patches. Cardiac rhabdomyomas and renal tumours (angiomyofibromas and renal cysts) may occur.
- Seizures are the most common presenting symptom (seen in up to 90%). Infants may present with infantile spasms. Early seizures correlate with significant learning difficulties.

FURTHER READING

O'Callaghan F. 2008: Tuberous sclerosis complex. *Paediatr Child Health;* 18: 30–36.
Umeoka S, Koyama T, Miki Y et al. 2008: Pictorial review of tuberous sclerosis in various organs. *RadioGraphics;* 28: e32; published online as 10.1148/rg.e32.

Case 24

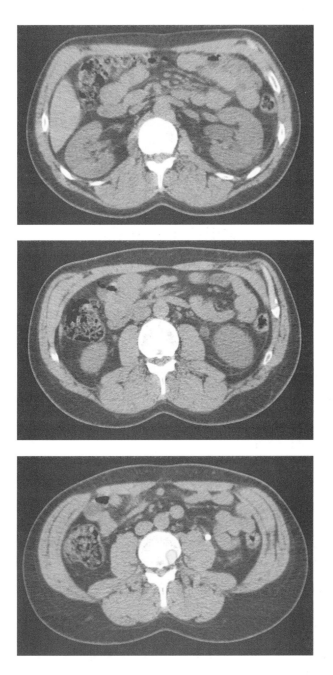

This 16-year-old male has left flank pain and haematuria.

1. What abnormalities are seen on the non-contrast CT scan of the abdomen?
2. What is the diagnosis?

ANSWERS

1. There is a left hydronephrosis, with dilatation of the left renal collecting system and proximal ureter. There is a high attenuation focus in the left ureter indicating a mid-ureteric calculus.
2. Left hydronephrosis secondary to an obstructing left ureteric calculus.

RADIOLOGY HOT LIST

- Non-contrast CT is now the gold standard in the investigation of renal calculi and renal tract obstruction in the adult population. It demonstrates almost all calcified stones (unlike plain films) without the possible complications associated with the intravenous contrast required for an IVU.
- Calculi are clearly visible as high-density foci, and their exact anatomical location can be ascertained using CT multi-planar reformats.
- Signs of renal tract obstruction include hydronephrosis, stranding of the perinephric and peri-ureteric fat, and ureteric dilatation to the level of the calculus.
- CT is performed judiciously in children due to the high radiation burden, and ultrasound remains the first-line test in the paediatric population. Small renal calculi may be difficult to see on ultrasound.

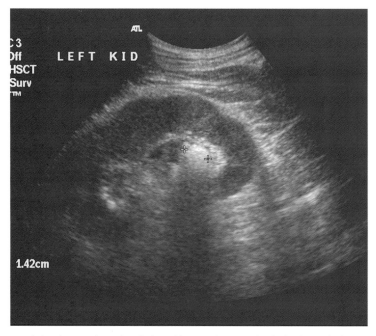

Renal ultrasound showing an echogenic calculus with posterior acoustic shadowing in the lower pole of the kidney.

CLINICAL HOT LIST

- Renal calculi are rare in children; they may be related to an underlying metabolic disorder (40%) or secondary to obstruction or infection. Associations also include congenital abnormalities of the renal tract, prematurity, prolonged immobility and urinary tract infection.
- The classical presentation of renal colic and macroscopic haematuria is uncommon in children. Calculi may be asymptomatic.
- Stones may be passed spontaneously or be removed by lithotripsy, cystoscopy or open surgery. Various types are as follows:

Stone type	Cause
Calcium stones	Hypercalcuria, hypercalcaemia secondary to hyperparathyroidism, excess vitamin D
Cystine stones	Cystinuria with renal tubular defect of amino acid transport
Oxalate stones	Primary hyperoxaluria, or secondary to small bowel disease and disordered absorption, e.g. Crohn's, post-surgical
Uric acid stones	Induction therapy for leukaemia

FURTHER READING

Coward RJM, Peters CJ, Duffy PG et al. 2003: Epidemiology of paediatric renal stone disease in the UK. *Arch Dis Child;* 88: 962–5.

Kraus SJ, Lebowitz RL, Royal SA. 1999: Renal calculi in children: imaging features that lead to diagnosis: a pictorial essay. *Pediatr Radiol;* 29: 624–30.

Case 25

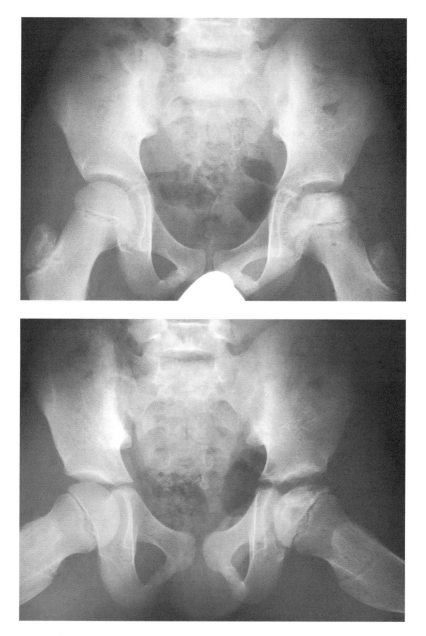

This 9-year-old boy presented to his GP with a 2-month history of left groin pain and intermittent limp. AP and frog-lateral pelvic X-rays were obtained.

1. What do they show?
2. What is the diagnosis?
3. What are the sequelae if untreated?

ANSWERS

1. There is flattening and sclerosis of the left femoral capital epiphysis with subchondral fissures.
2. Perthes disease (idiopathic avascular necrosis of the femoral head).
3. Abnormal bony remodelling with severe degenerative joint disease in early adulthood.

RADIOLOGY HOT LIST

- In the early phase the plain film is normal, but MRI will show bone marrow changes.

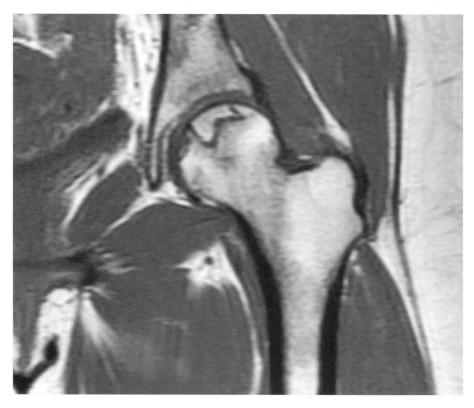

T1-weighted MRI shows a low signal serpiginous line within the left femoral head indicating acute avascular necrosis.

- Plain film changes reflect the healing process. A frog-lateral X-ray may be more sensitive than the AP view of the pelvis in demonstrating early changes.

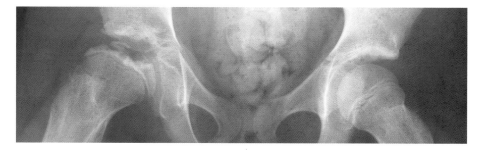

Late changes include a flattened misshapen femoral head with a short widened femoral neck.

CLINICAL HOT LIST

- Idiopathic avascular necrosis of the femoral head in childhood is due to interruption of the blood supply to the femoral epiphysis.
- It most commonly occurs in boys (4 : 1) aged between the ages of 4 and 10 years, and is bilateral in 10%. Frequency 1 : 1200 in those aged under 15 years.
- Clinical symptoms are gradual in onset with no recalled history of trauma. It may present with groin pain, limp, or limited hip movement.
- Treatment may include rest, traction, abduction bracing and osteotomy.
- Consider underlying pathology such as sickle cell disease, steroid therapy, and Gaucher's disease. Avascular necrosis can also occur secondary to trauma, infection, surgery and traction.

FURTHER READING

Gough-Palmer A, McHugh K. 2007: Investigating hip pain in a well child. *BMJ*; 334: 1216–7.

Case 26

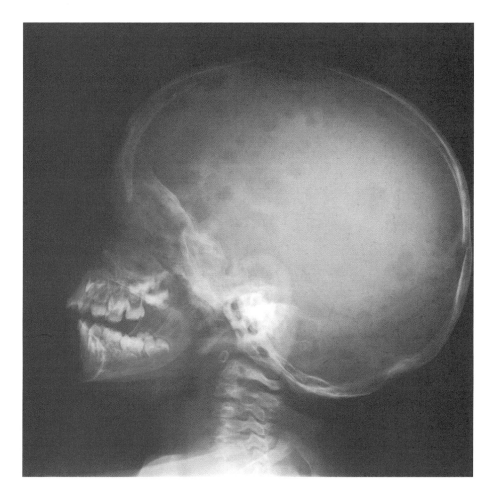

1. What abnormality is demonstrated on this lateral skull X-ray?
2. What is the most likely diagnosis?
3. What is the differential diagnosis?

ANSWERS

1. Well-defined, rounded lucent lesions are seen throughout the skull.
2. Langerhans' cell histiocytosis.
3. Bone metastases, most commonly from neuroblastoma or leukaemia.

RADIOLOGY HOT LIST

- The skull is the most common site for bone involvement in Langerhans' cell histiocytosis.
- The lesions are usually well defined and may have a sclerotic rim, giving a 'bevelled' edge appearance.
- The spine and ribs are also commonly involved. Radiological findings in the spine include lytic lesions and vertebral collapse (vertebra plana).

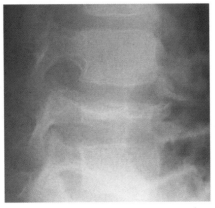

Lateral lumbar spine X-ray showing vertebra plana.

- Lytic lesions and periosteal reactions may be seen in the long bones.
- Extraskeletal disease may manifest radiologically as pulmonary interstitial infiltrates, cavitating nodules and pneumothorax.

CLINICAL HOT LIST

- Langerhans' cell histiocytosis is a disease of unknown aetiology with abnormal proliferation of phagocytic histiocytes. This may be an inflammatory or neoplastic process; there is evidence of immune dysregulation.
- There may be multisystem involvement, and the clinical course can vary from relatively benign to highly malignant and fatal.
- The disease process is variable and may involve the skin, lungs, bone marrow, lymphoreticular system (lymphadenopathy and hepatosplenomegaly), bone and the pituitary (diabetes insipidus).
- The treatment may include chemotherapy and radiotherapy.

FURTHER READING

Azouz EM, Saigal G, Rodriguez MM, Podda A. 2005: Langerhans' cell histiocytosis: pathology, imaging and treatment of skeletal involvement. *Pediatr Radiol;* 35: 103–15.

Case 27

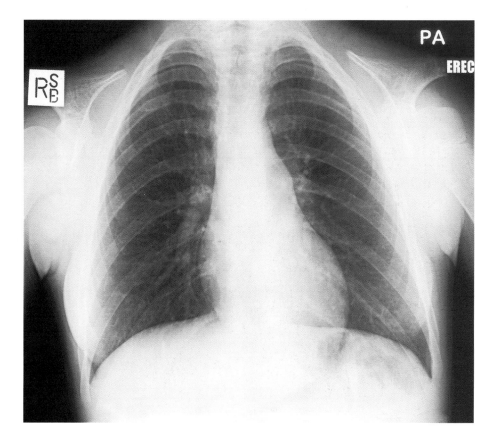

This 12-year-old girl had a chest infection when this X-ray was taken.

1. What abnormality is seen on the CXR?
2. What is the diagnosis?

ANSWERS

1. The clavicles are absent. The lungs are clear.
2. Cleidocranial dysostosis.

RADIOLOGY HOT LIST

- The clavicles may be hypoplastic or absent (10%).
- The chest may be narrow or bell shaped, with supernumerary ribs.
- The skull typically shows deficient ossification, widened sutures and fontanelles, and Wormian bones (small accessory bones within the sutures).

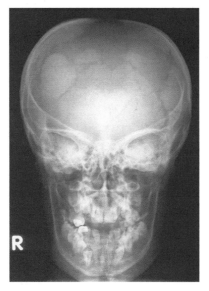

Skull X-ray showing multiple wormian bones and a big fontanelle.

CLINICAL HOT LIST

- Autosomal dominant disease with delayed/defective ossification of midline structures (particularly membranous bone).
- The characteristic features are:

Face	Hypoplastic maxilla, broad depressed bridge of nose, hypertelorism
Teeth	Delayed and abnormal dentition, malocclusion
Pelvis	Hypoplastic pubic rami, pubic diastasis
Hands	Long second metacarpal
Other features	Short stature, coxa vara

- Management requires orthopaedic and dental input.

FURTHER READING

Dighe M, Fligner C, Cheng E, Warren B, Dubinsky T. 2008: Fetal skeletal dysplasia: An approach to diagnosis with illustrative cases. *RadioGraphics;* 28: 1061–77.

Case 28

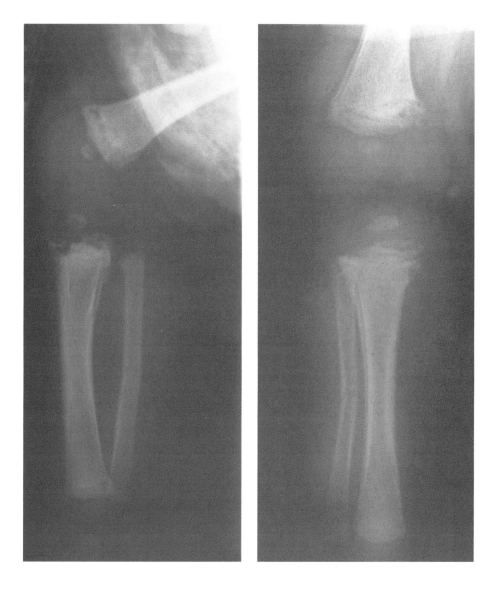

This 3-month-old baby presented to A & E with a history of inconsolable crying. On examination, he was not moving his right leg, which appeared to be swollen. His mother attributed this to an injury earlier in the week while changing his nappy.

1. What abnormalities are seen on the AP and lateral views of the right leg?
2. What is the most likely diagnosis?
3. What further investigations would you recommend?

ANSWERS

1. There are metaphyseal fractures of the distal right femur and proximal right tibia, with an exuberant callus response and periosteal reactions along the shaft of both bones. There is also a more recent fracture involving the midshaft of the right fibula.
2. NAI.
3. A full skeletal survey and a CT of the head.

RADIOLOGY HOT LIST

Radiological features suggestive of NAI include:

- Multiple fractures and fractures of different ages. The presence of a periosteal reaction indicates healing and is typically seen between 7 and 21 days following a fracture. Its absence usually indicates a more recent injury. Exaggerated callus formation is due to repetitive injury and/or a lack of treatment/immobilization.
- Any fracture without an appropriate explanation.
- Any fracture in a non-ambulant child.
- Metaphyseal fractures ('bucket-handle' or 'corner-chip'). These fractures are not usually seen in accidents and have a high specificity for NAI. These fractures may be subtle and meticulous radiography is required.

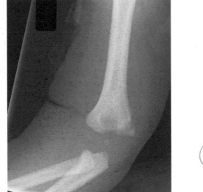

Metaphyseal fracture

Example of metaphyseal fracture.

- **Warning**: The initial plain film maybe normal—late films are essential if NAI is suspected. Bone scans may show abnormalities before the plain films.

FURTHER READING

Royal College of Radiologists and Royal College of Paediatrics and Child Health. 2008: Standards for Radiological Investigations of Suspected Non-accidental Injury.

Case 29

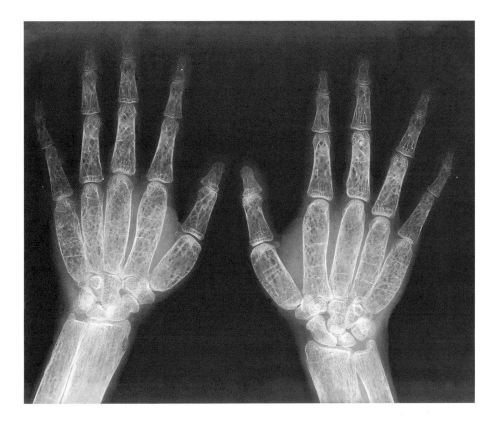

This 8-year-old Greek girl has chronic anaemia.

1. What does the X-ray of both hands show?
2. What is the likely diagnosis?

ANSWERS

1. There are widespread modelling abnormalities affecting all the bones of both hands, which show bony expansion, cortical thinning and a coarsened trabecular pattern. This implies marrow hyperplasia.
2. β-thalassaemia.

RADIOLOGY HOT LIST

- Marrow hyperplasia results in bony expansion and bony modelling abnormalities. This usually causes cortical thinning and a coarsened trabecular pattern.
- It also results in skull vault thickening and widening of the diploic space. The cortex of the inner and outer tables is progressively thinned and nearly invisible— if only the coarsened vertical trabeculations are seen, this leads to a 'hair-on-end' appearance. This is rarely seen nowadays.
- Involvement of the facial bones causes non-pneumatization of the paranasal air sinuses and mastoid air cells.
- Extramedullary haemopoiesis may cause a paravertebral mass on the CXR.

CLINICAL HOT LIST

- β-thalassaemia is a haemoglobinopathy caused by abnormal β-globin chain synthesis. It is commonly found in people of Mediterranean and Asian descent.
- It presents in the first year of life (when Hb A replaces Hb F). Features include anaemia, hepatosplenomegaly, recurrent fever and failure to thrive. Most children in the UK are diagnosed antenatally or as part of the newborn screening programme.
- Skeletal deformities may be prevented by a regular transfusion programme. Haemosiderosis may occur due to frequent transfusions and increased iron absorption. It can be prevented by iron chelation with desferrioxamine or the newer oral iron chelators.
- Bone marrow transplantation (BMT) is curative.

FURTHER READING

Davies HJ. 2007: Haemoglobinopathies. *Paediatr Child Health;* 17: 311–16.
Tunacı M, Tunacı A, Engin G et al. 1999: Imaging features of thalassemia. *Eur Radiol;* 9: 1894–1909.

Case 30

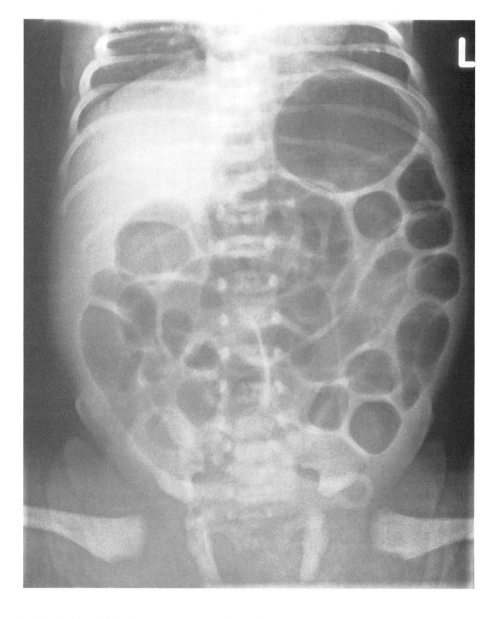

This 3-day-old baby was reviewed on the postnatal ward for failure to pass meconium. On examination the abdomen was distended with palpable bowel loops, and the anus appeared patent.

1. What does the plain AXR show?
2. What examination should be performed next?
3. What is the differential diagnosis?

ANSWERS

1. There are multiple loops of dilated gas-filled bowel within the distended abdomen. These appearances are in keeping with a low bowel obstruction.
2. A contrast enema.
3. The differential diagnosis of neonatal low bowel obstruction includes Hirschprung's disease, meconium ileus, functional immaturity (meconium plug syndrome), ileal and anorectal atresia.

RADIOLOGY HOT LIST

- Differentiating between small and large bowel obstruction is difficult in neonates. The presence of multiple loops of dilated gas-filled bowel usually indicates a low bowel obstruction. The presence of intra-peritoneal calcification indicates in-utero perforation, usually due to meconium ileus.
- A contrast enema is required to differentiate between the major causes of low bowel obstruction.
- In Hirschprung's disease, a contrast enema may delineate the transition zone between normal (innervated) dilated colon and the narrowed segment of aganglionic bowel, usually in the rectosigmoid region (short segment Hirschprung's disease). Total colonic Hirschprung's occurs in approximately 10% of cases and may be indistinguishable from meconium ileus (microcolon).

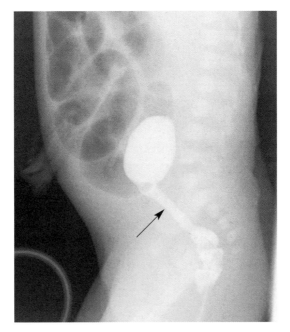

Contrast enema showing a rectosigmoid stricture due to Hirschprung's disease.

CLINICAL HOT LIST

- Pathology of Hirschsprung's disease: absent ganglia in both myenteric plexi (Auerbach and Meissner). The distribution is from the anus proximally, explained by a failure of caudal migration of neural crest cells.
- Presentation varies with length of affected bowel: 70% short segment, 20% long segment, 10% total colon (short segment may present as chronic severe constipation in the older child).
- The diagnosis is made by rectal biopsy. Management is surgical: either primary pull-through, or colostomy and delayed definitive procedure.
- 5% also have Down's syndrome.
- Complications include necrotizing enterocolitis (the risk persists even after surgery), perforation and failure to thrive.

FURTHER READING

Berrocal T, Lamas M, Gutiérrez J et al. 1999: Congenital anomalies of the small intestine, colon, and rectum. *RadioGraphics;* 19: 1219–36.
Swenson O. 2002: Hirschsprung's disease: A review. *Pediatrics;* 109: 914–18.

Case 31

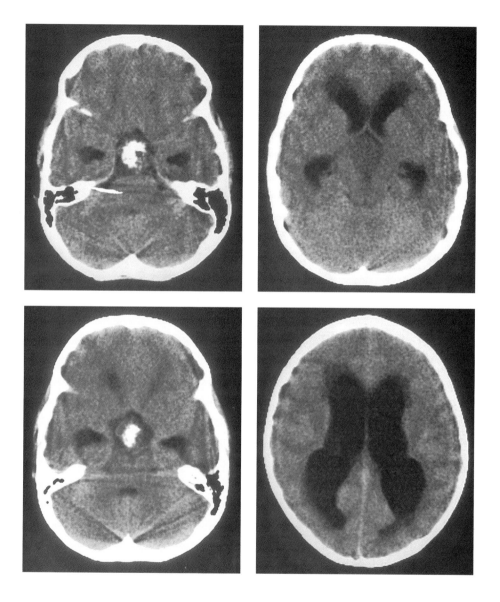

This 10-year-old boy was being investigated for headaches. On examination he was found to have a bitemporal hemianopia.

1. Describe two radiological abnormalities seen on the non-enhanced CT scan.
2. What is the diagnosis?

ANSWERS

1. There is a densely calcified suprasellar mass present. There is dilatation of the lateral ventricles (obstructive hydrocephalus). Periventricular low attenuation indicates acute hydrocephalus requiring urgent shunting.
2. Craniopharyngioma.

RADIOLOGY HOT LIST

- Skull X-rays may be normal, or show an enlarged or eroded pituitary fossa with associated calcification.

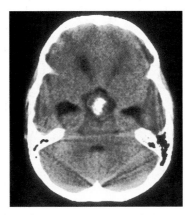

CT shows a cystic (75%) or mixed solid/cystic suprasellar mass, which is calcified in 70%. Large lesions may cause obstructive hydrocephalus.
- MRI exquisitely demonstrates the characteristic cystic component and local spread, e.g. involvement of optic chiasm and extension to hypothalamus or third ventricle.
- Scans should be performed in the postoperative period, to establish a baseline appearance for assessment of tumour recurrence.

CLINICAL HOT LIST

- Craniopharyngiomas are the commonest cause of a childhood suprasellar mass (median age of presentation 8 years). Despite being benign, slow-growing tumours they are nonetheless destructive.
- Presenting features include signs of raised intracranial pressure secondary to obstructive hydrocephalus, headache and visual field defects (classically bitemporal hemianopia).
- Endocrine dysfunction may occur as a result of abnormal levels of growth hormone, ACTH, TSH, TRH and ADH. The child may present with growth retardation or diabetes insipidus.
- Management is surgical resection, radiotherapy and endocrine replacement therapy.
- Long-term problems are common: learning difficulties, behavioural problems including hyperphagia, memory and vision disturbance and complex endocrinopathies. There is a 30% risk of recurrence.

FURTHER READING

Curran JG, O'Connor E. 2005: Imaging of craniopharyngioma. *Childs Nerv Syst;* 21: 635–9.
Williams T. 2004: Paediatric craniopharyngioma. *Arch Dis Child;* 89: 792.

Case 32

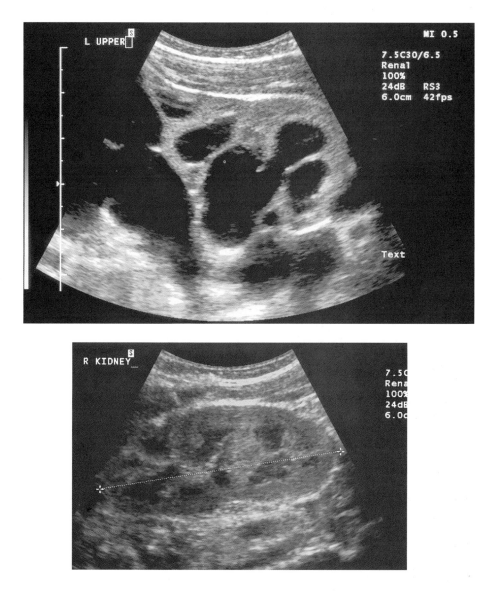

This 4-month-old girl is under investigation for a urinary tract infection. An USS of the kidneys was performed.

1. What does the ultrasound show?
2. What is the diagnosis?

ANSWERS

1. There is a duplex system on the left side, with marked dilatation of both the upper moiety and lower moiety PC systems. The right kidney is normal.
2. Duplex left kidney with an obstructed upper moiety. The lower moiety dilatation is due to reflux.

RADIOLOGY HOT LIST

- Ultrasound is the investigation of choice in delineating renal anatomy. It can demonstrate the obstructed upper moiety and may show a dilated ureter. Always consider the diagnosis where there is a 'cystic' lesion arising from the upper pole.
- The ureters may unite or have separate insertions. IVUs have traditionally been used to delineate ureteric anatomy, but CT urography is increasingly used in the adult population (it carries a high radiation burden).

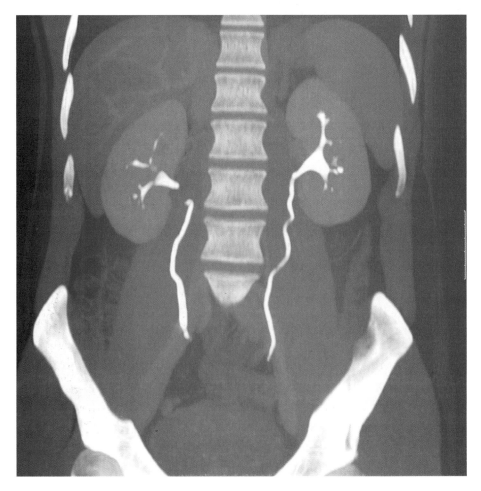

Normal CTU.

- MR urography (MRU) is an alternative non-radiation method of evaluating the ureters. Heavily T2-weighted images detect water content within the renal collecting system, spinal canal, biliary tree and some bowel loops. These are reformatted for optimum visualization of the renal upper tracts and bladder.

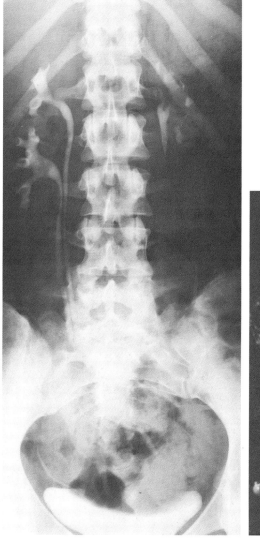

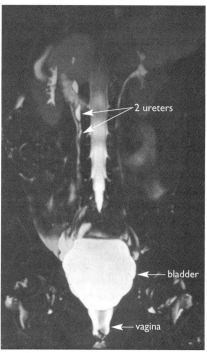

Traditional IVU depicting right renal duplex collecting system.

MRU depicting a right duplex collecting system and bladder. There is fluid in the vagina due to an ectopic right ureteric insertion.

- Classically the upper moiety has an ectopic insertion, usually into the bladder. There may be an associated ureterocele (seen as a filling defect in the bladder). The ectopic insertion makes the upper moiety prone to obstruction. Insertion into the bladder neck, urethra or vagina results in incontinence.

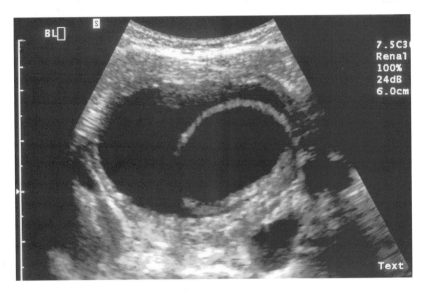

Ultrasound image of an ureterocele within the bladder.

- The lower moiety is prone to vesicoureteric reflux and renal scarring.

CLINICAL HOT LIST

- Duplication of the renal collecting system is the commonest congenital abnormality of the urinary tract. It is bilateral in 15–40%.
- Embryologically two separate ureteric buds associate with the mesonephric blastema (fetal nephrons).
- Most cases are asymptomatic and are an incidental finding. Some complete duplex kidneys are prone to obstruction, reflux and infection. The ectopic insertion of the upper moiety ureter can lead to incontinence in females.

FURTHER READING

Carrico C, Lebowitz RL. 1998: Incontinence due to an infrasphincteric ectopic ureter: why the delay in diagnosis and what the radiologist can do about it. *Pediatr Radiol*; 28: 942–9.

Williams H. 2007: Renal revision: from lobulation to duplication—what is normal? *Arch Dis Child Ed Pract*; 92: ep152–8.

Case 33

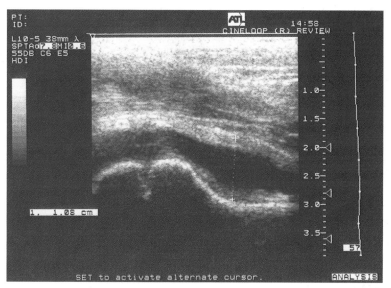

Right hip.

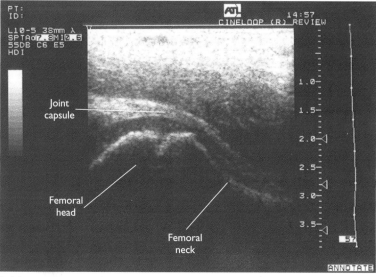

Left hip.

This 4-year-old boy presented to his GP with a 3-day history of fever and coryzal symptoms, and a 1-day history of right-sided limp. An ultrasound examination of his hips was performed.

1. What does the ultrasound show?
2. What is the most likely diagnosis?

ANSWERS

1. There is a joint effusion present in the right hip. The joint capsule is distended anteriorly with anechoic fluid lying between the capsule and the femoral neck. The left hip joint is normal.
2. Transient synovitis of the right hip (irritable hip), though a septic arthritis will need to be excluded.

RADIOLOGY HOT LIST

- Ultrasound is the examination of choice for the detection of a joint effusion. Comparison can be made between the normal and affected side.
- A complex effusion (containing internal echoes) is more suggestive of a septic arthritis. Simple fluid is anechoic on ultrasound, but this finding alone does not exclude a septic arthritis. Aspiration of fluid is required if a septic arthritis is suspected.
- Radiological evaluation of childhood limp should include an X-ray of the pelvis to look for bony pathology. Plain films are insensitive at detecting effusions, but large effusions may cause a relative increase in the medial joint space.

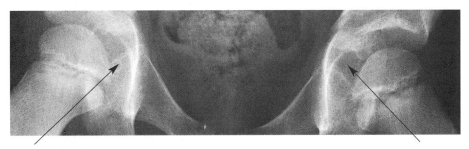

Normal joint   Increased joint space

CLINICAL HOT LIST

- Irritable hip occurs most commonly in boys aged 3–10 years. It usually follows a viral infection, presenting with sudden onset of hip pain and low-grade pyrexia. It is managed conservatively, with analgesia.
- The primary differential diagnosis is septic arthritis, when the child is usually systemically unwell and unable to weightbear. Serum inflammatory markers are usually raised, but the definitive test remains microbiological analysis of aspirated joint fluid.
- Causes of a joint effusion include transient synovitis, septic arthritis, trauma, juvenile idiopathic arthritis, and early Perthes disease.
- Hip pathology may present with referred knee pain. Always examine the hip!

FURTHER READING

Beresford MW, Cleary AG. 2005: Evaluation of a limping child. *Curr Paed;* 15: 15–22.
Do TT. 2000: Transient synovitis as a cause of painful limps in children. *Curr Opin Pediatr;* 12:48–51.

Case 34

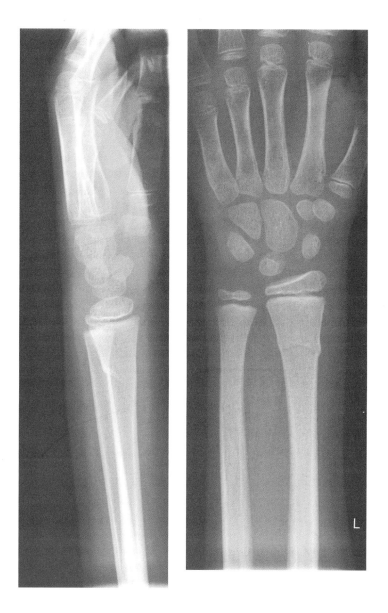

This 5-year-old boy attended A & E after a fall whilst playing.

1. What abnormality is seen on the plain radiograph of the left wrist?
2. What is the diagnosis?

ANSWERS

1. There is buckling of the cortex with a faint transverse lucency seen in the distal radius.
2. Torus fracture of the distal radius.

RADIOLOGY HOT LIST

- The cortex of a bone is normally a smooth, unbroken line.
- Impaction results in cortical buckling and a torus fracture (torus is derived from the Latin word meaning protruberance or bulge).
- A greenstick fracture (less common) occurs if the bone is angulated beyond its capacity for bending, leading to a fracture on the convex side of the bend. Muscular spasm may then hold the fracture open at this 'hinge' point.

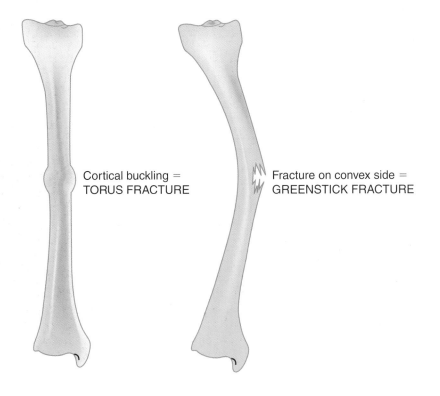

Cortical buckling =
TORUS FRACTURE

Fracture on convex side =
GREENSTICK FRACTURE

CLINICAL HOT LIST

- Torus fractures are treated with immobilization and pain relief.
- Greenstick fractures with pronounced angulation may require reduction and correct positioning prior to immobilization and healing.

Case 35

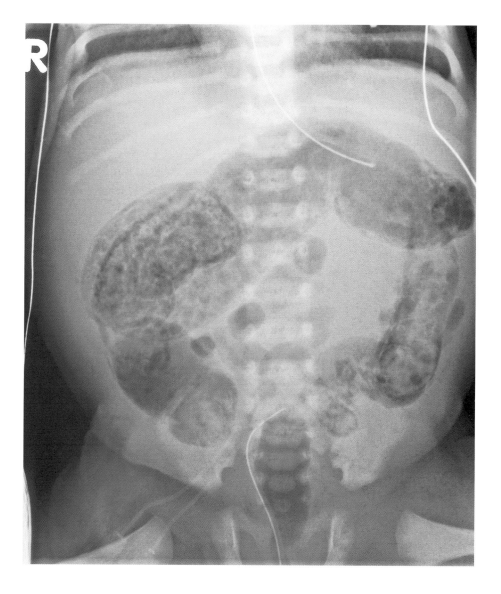

A 7-day-old baby, born at 29 weeks gestation, is noted to be pale and lethargic on the neonatal unit.

1. What radiological sign is seen on the plain abdominal radiograph?
2. What is the diagnosis?
3. Give four possible risk factors for this condition.

ANSWERS

1. There are lucencies within the bowel wall, representing intramural gas (pneumatosis intestinalis). There is no evidence of perforation, or gas within the portal venous system.
2. Necrotizing enterocolitis (NEC).
3. Risk factors include prematurity, intrauterine growth retardation, perinatal asphyxia, hypoxia and shock, sepsis, polycythaemia, umbilical catheterization and hypertonic feeds.

RADIOLOGY HOT LIST

- The initial plain film may be normal. Early radiological signs include dilated loops of bowel and bowel wall thickening. The colon and terminal ileum are most commonly affected.
- Intramural gas is characteristic of NEC, and may appear as linear lucencies or 'foamy' collections of gas.
- Search for free air, which may appear as a central lucency overlying the abdomen (as the baby is supine), or outlining the falciform ligament (which appears as a linear density in the midline or right upper quadrant).
- Look for portal venous gas (linear lucencies within the liver that extend peripherally).

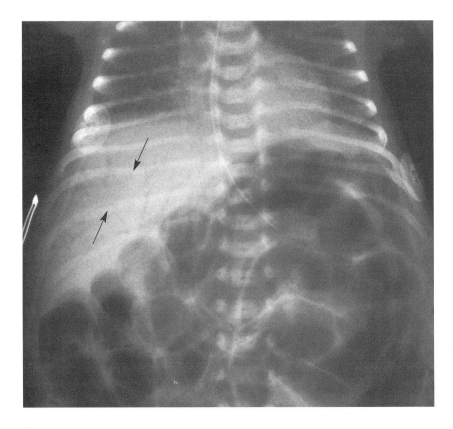

CLINICAL HOT LIST

- It is primarily a condition of preterm and low birthweight babies whose immature gut is vulnerable to a variety of insults, which manifest as NEC.
- Cardinal mechanisms are gut hypoperfusion and ischaemia, though an infective process is also implicated.
- Clinical presentation ranges from systemic features (lethargy, hypotonia, shock and apnoea) to abdominal distension, bilious vomiting and rectal bleeding.
- Management of NEC may be medical (resuscitation, systemic support, total parenteral nutrition, antibiotics) and/or surgical (peritoneal drainage, laparotomy, resection). Late complications include intestinal stricture (20%) and short gut syndrome (postsurgical resection).

FURTHER READING

Coombs RC. 2003: The prevention and management of necrotizing enterocolitis. *Curr Paed;* 13: 184–9.

Epelman M, Daneman A, Navarro OM et al. 2007: Necrotizing enterocolitis: Review of state-of-the-art imaging findings with pathologic correlation. *RadioGraphics;* 27: 285–305.

Case 36

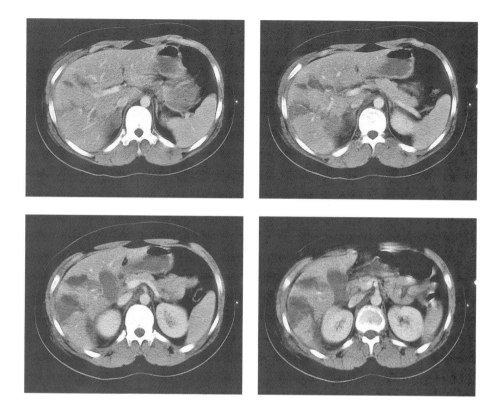

This 13-year-old boy was involved in a road traffic accident, and complained of right upper quadrant pain.

1. What does the contrast-enhanced CT scan of the abdomen show?
2. What is the diagnosis?

ANSWERS

1. There are multiple, irregular, low-attenuation areas within the right lobe of the liver. The intrahepatic vessels are normally opacified. No free fluid is present.
2. Multiple liver lacerations with haematomas secondary to blunt trauma.

RADIOLOGY HOT LIST

- Liver lacerations are typically branching or rounded low-attenuation areas.
- Haematomas usually appear as poorly defined areas of low attenuation. High-attenuation areas may represent active haemorrhage.
- A subcapsular haematoma usually has a lenticular or crescent-shaped configuration.
- Look for free fluid (haemoperitoneum) and other visceral injuries. There is an associated splenic injury in 45%.

CLINICAL HOT LIST

- The liver is the second most frequently injured intra-abdominal viscus (after the spleen) in blunt trauma. The right lobe is most commonly affected.
- Following blunt abdominal trauma, raised liver enzymes are an indication to perform an abdominal CT in the haemodynamically stable child.
- Liver trauma is usually managed conservatively (in > 90% children). Embolization or surgery is indicated for continued bleeding.
- Complications occur in up to 20% (delayed rupture, haemobilia, infected haematoma, arteriovenous fistula).

FURTHER READING

McBride J, Knight D, Piper J et al. 2005: *Advanced Paediatric Life Support: The Practical Approach* (4th ed.) London: Blackwell Publishing.

Yoon W, Jeong YY, Kim JK et al. 2005: CT in blunt liver trauma. *RadioGraphics;* 25: 87–104.

Case 37

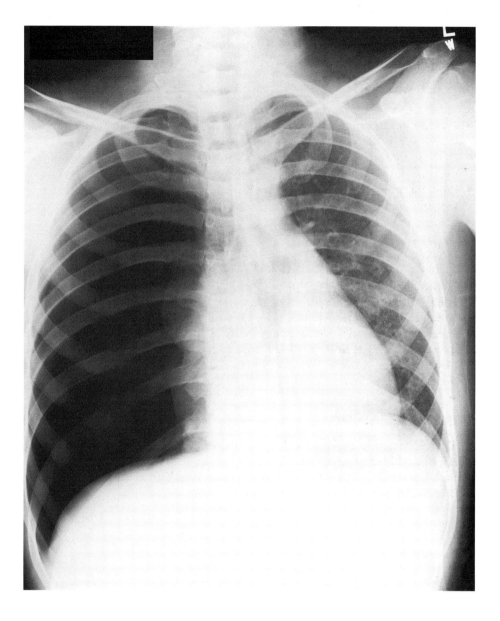

This 16-year-old male presented to A & E with an acute onset of dyspnoea and pleuritic chest pain.

1. What does the CXR show?
2. What is the diagnosis?

ANSWERS

1. The right hemithorax is hyperlucent with complete absence of pulmonary markings. The right hemidiaphragm is depressed and the mediastinum is displaced to the left.
2. Right tension pneumothorax.

RADIOLOGY HOT LIST

- Always assess the pulmonary vascularity when considering unequal lucency on the CXR—is it normal, reduced (implying abnormal lung), or absent (pneumothorax)?
- Look for a free lung edge. Mediastinal shift and/or a depressed diaphragm indicate the presence of a tension pneumothorax.
- Other causes of a unilateral hyperlucent hemithorax include patient rotation, air trapping (e.g. secondary to a foreign body, congenital lobar emphysema), reduced pulmonary perfusion and chest wall abnormalities.

CLINICAL HOT LIST

- Childhood pneumothorax is associated with trauma, asthma, cystic fibrosis, pulmonary infections (including tuberculosis), Marfan's syndrome and mechanical ventilation.
- Treatment options include observation, simple aspiration and chest drain insertion. The choice will depend on clinical presentation and severity.
- Life-threatening tension pneumothorax needs immediate intervention—do not wait for an X-ray!

FURTHER READING

McBride J, Knight D, Piper J et al. 2005: *Advanced Paediatric Life Support: The Practical Approach* (4th ed.) London: Blackwell Publishing.
Sjirk J, Westra E, Wallace C. 2005: Imaging evaluation of pediatric chest trauma. *Radiol Clin N Am;* 43: 267–81.

Case 38

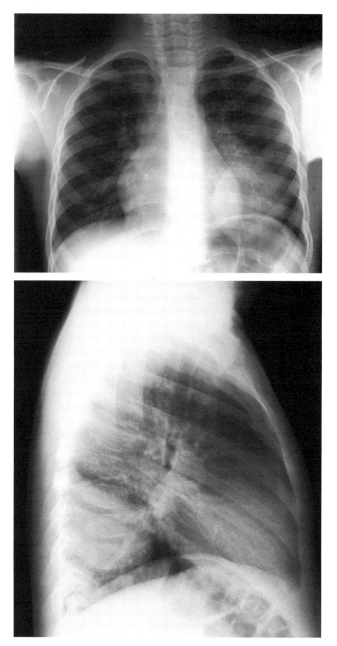

A 3-year-old girl was admitted via A & E with fever and cough. On examination she is pyrexial, with tachypnoea and tachycardia.

1. What abnormality is seen on the AP and lateral CXR?
2. What is the most likely diagnosis?

ANSWERS

1. There is a rounded opacity in the left lower lobe, which is intrapulmonary, and clearly separated from the spine. There is no air–fluid level or rib erosion.
2. Left lower lobe round pneumonia.

RADIOLOGY HOT LIST

- Round pneumonia is the most common cause of an apparent mass lesion in the paediatric chest. In the appropriate clinical setting a follow-up CXR after antibiotic therapy is the most pragmatic approach. With time, the initially round pneumonia develops into a more typical consolidation before eventual resolution.
- The lesion is clearly not paravertebral, making neurogenic tumours, a paraspinal abscess or extramedullary haematopoiesis unlikely.
- Other causes of solitary lung nodules:

Congenital	Bronchogenic cyst, lung sequestration, arteriovenous malformation, bronchial atresia
Infection	Abscess, granuloma
Tumour	Metastases (e.g. Wilms tumour), primary lung tumour: primitive neuroectodermal tumour (PNET), pulmonary blastoma

CLINICAL HOT LIST

- Round pneumonia is usually seen in the early consolidative phase of pneumococcal pneumonia.

FURTHER READING

Kim YM, Donnelly LF. 2007: Round pneumonia: imaging findings in a large series of children. *Pediatr Radiol;* 37:1235–40. Epub 2007 Oct 19.

Case 39

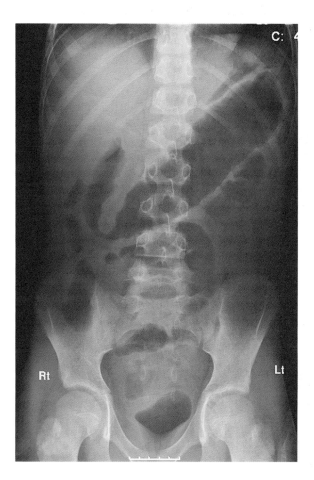

This 13-year-old boy has a 6-week history of abdominal pain and bloody diarrhoea. He has lost a considerable amount of weight. On examination, he has generalized abdominal tenderness. An AXR has been performed.

1. What does the AXR show?
2. What is the diagnosis?
3. What possible complications may occur?

ANSWERS

1. The abdominal film shows a central distended featureless loop of bowel, which represents bowel wall thickening within the dilated transverse colon. There is loss of the normal colonic haustral folds, causing thumb-printing. The colon is empty, with no formed faecal residue present.
2. Acute colitis, in this case due to ulcerative colitis.
3. Complications include toxic megacolon, perforation and abscess formation.

RADIOLOGY HOT LIST

- Most children with acute colitis do not require intensive imaging. The plain film may show a generalized absence of faecal residue, with a variable bowel gas pattern. Severe bowel wall thickening may be evident as 'thumb-printing', due to severe swelling of the normally thin colonic haustra. Toxic megacolon occurs if there is marked dilatation of the diseased colon. This requires careful X-ray follow-up, as there is significant risk of perforation if the colon is markedly distended.
- Ultrasound may demonstrate bowel wall thickening, surrounding inflammation, free fluid and localized collections. It may miss small perforations as free air may be missed.
- CT is useful to exclude small or sealed perforations, to delineate the extent of the colitis, to identify abscess formation and guide drainage procedures.

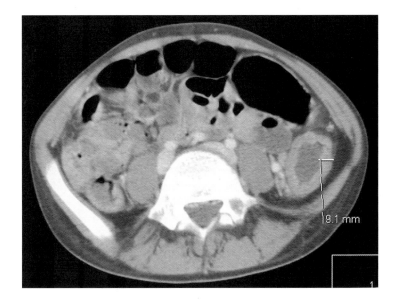

The normal colonic wall usually measures < 3 mm. The descending colon is fluid filled, and shows circumferential wall thickening, indicating colitis.

CLINICAL HOT LIST

- 25% of inflammatory bowel disease presents in childhood and this is increasing; the aetiology is unknown (genetic predisposition, environment, immune dysfunction, role of infection).
- Classically ulcerative colitis presents with bloody diarrhoea, abdominal pain and weight loss; the differential is wide but infection must be excluded.
- Diagnosis is confirmed with endoscopy and biopsy.
- Treatment aims to induce and then maintain remission, with attention to growth, nutrition and development. Options include corticosteroids (at diagnosis and for flares), 5ASA derivatives, and immunosuppression, e.g. with azathioprine. Surgery may be required for failure of medical management.
- Toxic dilatation of the colon is a life-threatening emergency, requiring medical and surgical input. Management includes fluid resuscitation, transfusion, intravenous steroids and antibiotics, frequent review and abdominal imaging (AXR, ultrasound). Up to 50% with toxic megacolon will require surgery.

FURTHER READING

Allan RA. 2001: Imaging in inflammatory bowel disease. *Imaging;* 13: 272–84.
Beattie RM, Croft NM, Fell JM, Afzal NA, Heuschkel RB. 2006: Inflammatory bowel disease. *Arch Dis Child;* 91: 426–32.

Case 40

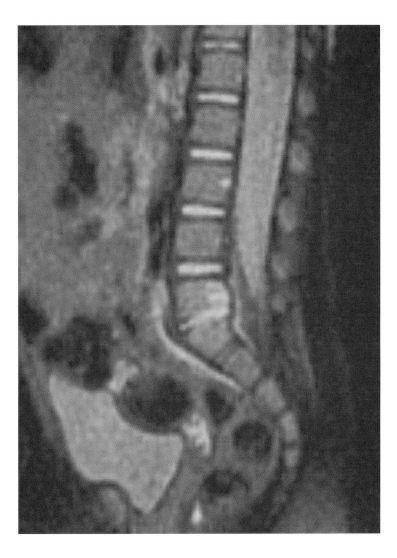

This 11-month-old boy has refused to walk for 2 weeks and appears to be in pain. He is apyrexial, but has raised inflammatory markers. An MRI scan of the lumbar spine has been performed.

1. What does the MRI scan show?
2. What is the diagnosis?

ANSWERS

1. There is high signal in the L5–S1 disc, which is contiguous with increased signal in the adjacent L5 vertebral body. There is destruction of both vertebral end-plates, and there is bulging of the posterior vertebral margin of L5.
2. Discitis of the L5–S1 disc with associated osteomyelitis of the L5 vertebra.

RADIOLOGY HOT LIST

- The normal intervertebral discs show moderately high signal on T2-weighted MRI. In discitis, there is alteration in the disc signal (either loss of signal, or exaggerated high signal) and loss of disc height.
- There may be signal alteration in the adjacent vertebral bodies related to bone marrow oedema, which is best seen at the end-plates that directly abut the discs.
- Plain films may show loss of disc height with erosion of the adjacent vertebral end-plates. Bone scans show intense tracer uptake at the site of inflammation.
- MRI is the modality of choice in the assessment of discitis. It can easily assess early inflammation in the disc and vertebral bodies, whilst identifying complications such as epidural abscesses, which may require urgent drainage.

CLINICAL HOT LIST

- Inflammation is secondary to infection of the vertebral disc space. Haematogenous spread of infection is most common, as the disc space remains vascular in childhood. Unlike in adults, a primary site of infection is unusual.
- *Staph. aureus* is the commonest organism and may be identified in blood culture or by direct aspirate.
- Presentation is typically in a child aged younger than 4 years with sudden onset of back pain, fever and refusal to walk.
- Management includes IV antibiotics, bed rest and occasionally decompressive surgery.
- There is usually complete recovery; sometimes vertebral fusion is seen.

FURTHER READING

Brown R, Hussain M, McHugh K et al. 2001: Discitis in young children. *J Bone Joint Surg Br;* 83: 106–11.

Soroosh Mahboubi M, Morris C. 2001: Imaging of spinal infections in children. *Radiol Clin N Am;* 39: 215–22.

Case 41

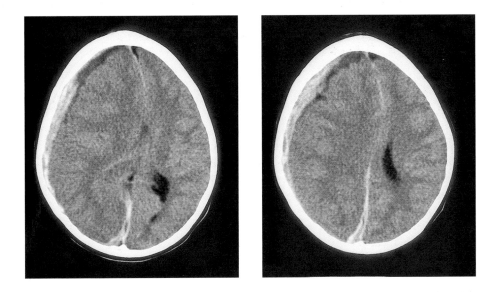

This 1-year-old girl was brought to A & E after a sudden collapse at home. On examination she was unresponsive to pain with bradycardia.

1. Name three abnormalities seen on the non-enhanced CT scan of the head.
2. What is the diagnosis?
3. What is the most likely underlying cause?

ANSWERS

1. There is midline shift and effacement of the right lateral ventricle. There is a right subdural collection with areas of high and low attenuation within it. A further high-attenuation subdural collection is seen posteriorly, along the interhemispheric fissure, adjacent to the falx cerebri.
2. Acute chronic right subdural haematoma and acute interhemispheric fissure subdural haematoma. There has been significant head trauma.
3. Non-accidental injury (NAI).

RADIOLOGY HOT LIST

- Subdural collections appear as crescent shaped, often extending widely across the convexity of a cerebral hemisphere.
- Fresh blood usually appears initially as high density, becomes isodense with brain after 7–10 days, and low density after 3–4 weeks.
- Features of subdural haematomas that are suspicious for NAI:
  — Subdural haematoma with no associated skull fracture, implying shaking injury.
  — Bilateral subdurals.
  — Subdurals of different ages (areas of high and low attenuation).
  — Acute interhemispheric fissure subdural or falx haemorrhage (bright irregularly thickened falx).
  — Subdurals in the presence of retinal haemorrhages, implying acceleration/deceleration force.

CLINICAL HOT LIST

	Acute subdural	Chronic subdural
Time of injury	< 3 days	> 3 weeks
Presentation	Shock, raised intracranial pressure, cerebral oedema	Insidious, few clinical signs, no raised intracranial pressure
Outcome	50% mortality. Survivors have high risk of severe neurological deficit	80% full recovery

- Subdural haematoma is uncommon in accidental head injury but usually present in most fatal head injuries caused by NAI.
- The mechanism of injury is rotation of the brain within the fixed cranial vault and dura, causing tearing of the bridging veins. Associated retinal haemorrhages are present in up to 70%.
- Neurosurgical consultation is mandatory, with intensive care management of raised intracranial pressure (in an acute presentation).
- All cases of suspected NAI require detailed clinical examination, documentation of all injuries, fundoscopy, skeletal survey and involvement of the child protection team.

FURTHER READING

Datta S, Stoodley N, Jayawant S, Renowden S, Kemp A. 2005: Neuroradiological aspects of subdural haemorrhages. *Arch Dis Child;* 90: 947–51.

Rao P, Carty H. 1999: Non-accidental radiology: review of the radiology. *Clin Radiol;* 54: 11–24.

Case 42

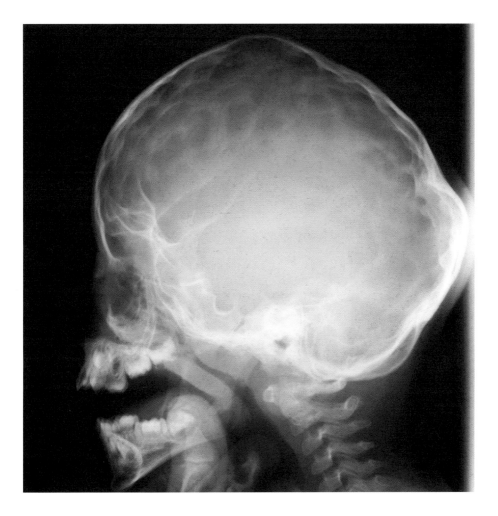

This 2-year-old boy has developmental delay.

1. What does the lateral skull X-ray show?
2. What is the diagnosis?

ANSWERS

1. The skull is microcephalic and has an abnormal shape. The normal sagittal, coronal and lambdoid sutures are obliterated (fused). There is a 'copper-beaten' appearance to the skull due to prominent convolutional markings on the inner table.
2. Craniosynostosis with raised intracranial pressure.

RADIOLOGY HOT LIST

- Craniosynostosis refers to premature closure of one or more skull sutures, leading to an abnormally shaped skull.
- The sagittal suture is best seen on the frontal view, whilst the lambdoid suture is best seen on the lateral view. The coronal suture should be visible on both views.
- Involvement of individual sutures gives rise to characteristic deformities, e.g. premature fusion of the sagittal suture results in scaphocephaly.
- If all three sutures are involved, raised intracranial pressure may result, manifesting as the 'copper-beaten' skull. (This appearance can be normal before the age of 6 months.)

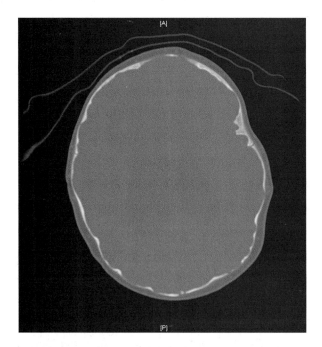

CT brain (bone windows) showing scalloping of the inner table of the skull due to raised intracranial pressure, which causes the copper beaten skull appearance.

CLINICAL HOT LIST

- Craniosynostosis may be primary or secondary; the causes of the latter are as follows:

Causes of secondary craniosynostosis	Examples
Syndromes (associated with syndactyly and polysyndactyly)	Apert, Carpenter, Crouzon, Pfieffer, clover leaf skull
Haematological	Sickle cell anaemia, thalassaemia
Metabolic	Rickets, hypercalcaemia, hyperthyroidism
Bone dysplasia	Hypophosphatasia, achondroplasia, metaphyseal dysplasia
Microcephaly	Brain atrophy/dysgenesis
Postsurgical	Post-shunting procedures

- Presentation may be with an abnormal head shape, symptoms of raised intracranial pressure (e.g. irritability, vomiting, headache, seizures and developmental delay) or exophthalmos.
- Neurosurgical intervention is indicated for raised intracranial pressure, progressive exophthalmos, or those at high risk of developing these complications. Cosmetic correction should only be contemplated for severe deformity.

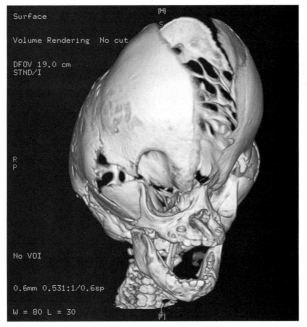

3D volume-rendered image of Pfieffer syndrome, with fusion of the coronal suture, and a widely separated sagittal suture.

FURTHER READING

Glass RBJ, Fernbach SK, Norton KI, Choi PS, Naidich TP. 2004: The infant skull: A vault of information. *RadioGraphics;* 24: 507–22.

Case 43

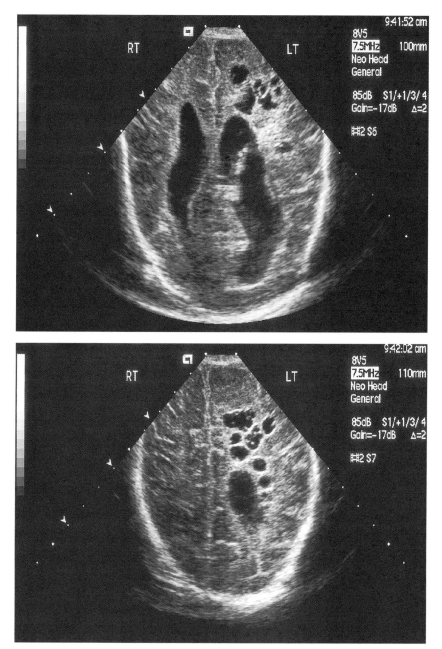

This baby was born at 28 weeks' gestation. This cranial ultrasound was performed at 4 weeks of age.

1. What does the ultrasound show?
2. What is the diagnosis?

ANSWERS

1. There is bilateral ventricular dilatation, with periventricular cystic change within the deep white matter of the left parietal lobe. The surrounding parenchyma is also of increased echogenicity.
2. Periventricular leucomalacia (PVL).

RADIOLOGY HOT LIST

- The earliest sign of PVL on cranial ultrasound is increased periventricular echogenicity. However this can be a normal finding in neonates, so the diagnosis may be missed if changes are subtle. Changes are often bilateral but asymmetrical.
- Cavitation occurs 1–6 weeks after the ischaemic insult, with small cystic spaces seen adjacent to the ventricles. There may be associated cerebral atrophy and ventriculomegaly.
- MRI is sensitive (and superior to cranial ultrasound) in the acute, subacute and chronic phases of PVL. The severity of changes on MRI is well correlated with neurologic outcomes such as cerebral palsy, visual impairment and delayed motor development.

CLINICAL HOT LIST

- Periventricular leucomalacia occurs after an ischaemic insult to the premature brain, which leads to tissue necrosis.
- Ischaemic infarction occurs at the watershed zone between the central and peripheral vascular supply. The watershed area between the different vascular territories lies in the periventricular region in preterm infants, unlike full-term infants, in whom it is located in the cortical and subcortical region.
- The prognosis is variable, ranging from mild intellectual impairment/ developmental delay to audiovisual deficit, epilepsy, cerebral palsy and microcephaly. Generalized PVL results in neurological deficit in nearly 100% of cases. Spastic diplegia or quadriplegia is more likely to be associated with this type of lesion.

FURTHER READING

Epelman M, Daneman A, Blaser SI et al. 2006: Differential diagnosis of intracranial cystic lesions at head US: Correlation with CT and MR imaging. *RadioGraphics;* 26: 173–96.
Levene M. 2005: The sequelae of periventricular haemorrhage. *Curr Paed;* 15: 375–80.

Case 44

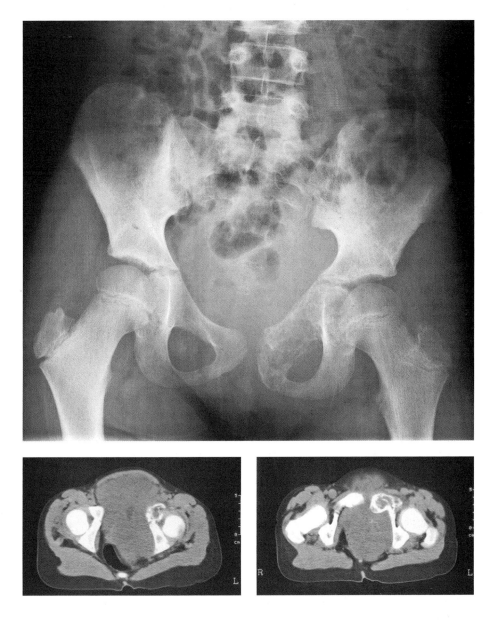

This 7-year-old girl presented with left-sided limp and groin pain. An X-ray of the pelvis was requested, followed by a CT scan.

1. What does the plain film show?
2. What additional information is on the CT?
3. What is the diagnosis?

ANSWERS

1. The left superior pubic ramus is expanded, with an ill-defined and permeative abnormality of the bone texture. The left proximal femur is osteopenic, probably due to disuse osteoporosis.
2. There is an associated non-ossified soft tissue mass in the left hemipelvis, displacing the rectum to the right.
3. Ewing's sarcoma of the left superior pubic ramus.

RADIOLOGY HOT LIST

- Ewing's sarcoma occurs in the long bones in 60% (most commonly the femur and tibia) and in the flat bones in 40% (pelvis and ribs).
- Plain films classically show a permeative, ill-defined lytic lesion with an associated soft tissue mass. There may be a periosteal reaction (classically lamellar 'onion-peel' but can also be spiculated 'sun-burst' pattern).

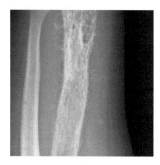

Sun-burst periosteal reaction.

- MRI will assess the extent of marrow involvement and local extra-osseous disease. Chest CT is required for the detection of pulmonary metastases, while a bone scan will detect skeletal metastases.
- Overlap occurs in the radiological appearances of Ewing's sarcoma and osteosarcoma. Infection and eosinophilic granuloma can occasionally give similar appearances on the plain film and a bone biopsy is required in all cases to establish histology.

CLINICAL HOT LIST

- Ewing's sarcoma is a rare malignant bone tumour of primitive small round cells. The peak incidence is 10–15 years (> 60% occur in the second decade of life). It presents with painful swelling at the affected site. Systemic symptoms may indicate metastatic disease.
- Features associated with a poor prognosis include metastases at diagnosis, proximal site (e.g. pelvis), soft tissue involvement and poor response to chemotherapy.
- Treatment consists of intensive chemotherapy followed by either surgery or radiotherapy.
- The long-term survival rate is 60% without metastases, < 25% with metastases.

FURTHER READING

Grier HE. 1997: The Ewing family of tumors. *Pediatr Clin North Am;* 44: 991–1004.
Miller SL, Hoffer FA. 2001: Malignant and benign bone tumors. *Radiol Clin N Am;* 39: 673–99.

Case 45

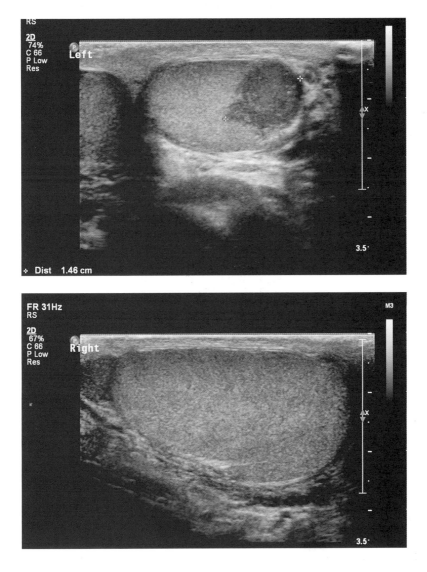

This 17-year-old teenager noticed a hard, non-tender swelling of his left testis.

1. What scan has been performed?
2. What does it show?
3. What is the diagnosis?

ANSWERS

1. An USS of the scrotum.
2. There is a low-density focal mass in the lower pole of the left testis. The right testis is normal.
3. Left-sided testicular tumour.

RADIOLOGY HOT LIST

- Testes have a uniform homogeneous echotexture on ultrasound, so any focal lesion in a teenager or young adult should be regarded with suspicion—it probably represents a tumour.
- Epididymo-orchitis usually results in a generalized increase in size of the testis and epididymis, which may appear echopoor or heterogeneous, with increased vascularity.
- Germ cell tumours (GCTs) are the most common tumour.
- A USS of the abdomen and pelvis should also be performed as the lymphatic drainage is via the intra-abdominal para-aortic nodes.
- Confirmed cases require formal staging with CT of the chest, abdomen and pelvis.

CLINICAL HOT LIST

- The treatment of a suspicious testicular mass is inguinal orchidectomy.
- Testicular GCTs are rare (incidence approximately 7.5 : 100,000).
- GCT is the most common tumour in men aged 20–30 years. GCTs are subdivided into seminoma and teratoma.
- 97% have a palpable lump at presentation, 31% have pain, and 10% have a history of recent trauma.
- Hydrocoeles and gynaecomastia are rare presentations.
- 75% have raised tumour markers (AFP, HCG and LDH) at presentation.
- Seminomas and teratomas have different clinical outcomes and require different clinical management.
- Following histopathological confirmation, treatment options include: surveillance, chemotherapy and/or radiotherapy depending upon histology, vascular and lymphatic invasion and radiological staging.

FURTHER READING

Scottish Intercollegiate Guidelines Network. 1998: Management of adult testicular germ cell tumours. A National Clinical Guideline.

Case 46

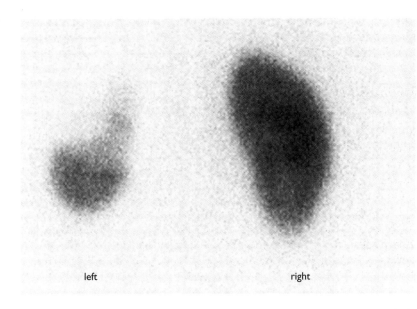

left   right

This study was obtained on a 10-year-old girl under investigation for hypertension. An abdominal ultrasound had demonstrated a small left kidney but no other significant abnormality.

1. What is the examination?
2. What does it show?

ANSWERS

1. This is a technetium-99m DMSA scan.
2. The left kidney is small, with very poor tracer uptake (cold spots) in the upper pole and reduced uptake in the lower pole. The appearance is consistent with renal scarring. The right kidney appears to be normal.

RADIOLOGY HOT LIST

- DMSA is taken up in the proximal convoluted tubules, with minimal renal excretion. It accumulates in the renal cortex. Reduced uptake indicates areas of scarring (cortical loss). The relative amount of uptake by each kidney reflects differential function.
- DMSA scan is the investigation of choice for assessing renal scarring, which can be missed on an ultrasound investigation. (For further discussion see 'Rules and tools'.)

CLINICAL HOT LIST

- Blood pressure (BP) gradually increases through childhood, with most people following a constant percentile. Early childhood hypertension (> 95th percentile) usually has an underlying cause. Essential hypertension rarely occurs before adolescence (make sure an appropriately sized paediatric BP cuff has been used!)
- Hypertension may be asymptomatic or cause headaches, blurred vision, heart failure, stroke, seizures and coma.
- Causes of childhood hypertension are:

Renal	Dysplastic kidney, polycystic disease, obstructive uropathy, reflux nephropathy
Endocrine	Neuroblastoma, phaeochromocytoma, congenital adrenal hyperplasia, Cushing's syndrome, hyperaldosteronism
Vascular	Aortic coarctation, renal artery stenosis, renal vein thrombosis, arteritis
Neurological	Raised intracranial pressure, encephalitis

- Usual investigations include serum electrolytes and creatinine, urinanalysis, plasma and urine hormone/amine levels, and renal ultrasound.
- Treatment options are directed towards both the underlying cause and maintaining normal blood pressure. Hypertension can be controlled by a combination of diuretics, β-blockers, angiotensin-converting enzyme (ACE) inhibitors, calcium channel blockers and vasodilators. The prognosis depends on the underlying cause.

FURTHER READING

Mitsnefes MM. 2006: Hypertension in children and adolescents. *Paediatr Clin N Am;* 53: 493–512.

Robuck D. 2008: Childhood hypertension: what does the radiologist contribute? *Pediatr Radiol;* 30: 501–7.

Case 47

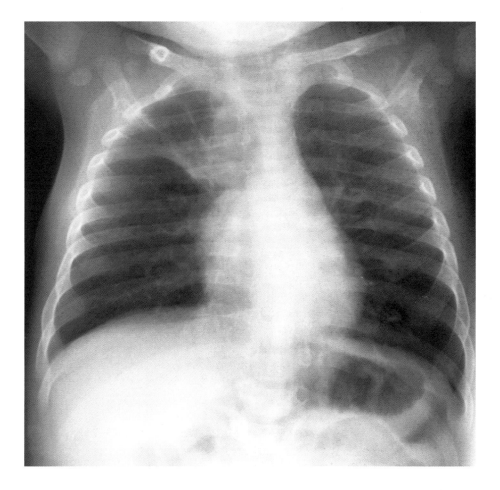

This 6-month-old girl was seen in A & E with fever and wheeze. On examination she had tachypnoea, intercostal recession and widespread wheeze on auscultation.

1. What does the CXR show?
2. What is the diagnosis?

ANSWERS

1. The lungs are hyperinflated. There is partial collapse of the right upper lobe (elevation of the horizontal fissure).
2. Bronchiolitis.

RADIOLOGY HOT LIST

- The CXR in bronchiolitis may be normal.
- The commonest abnormality is hyperinflation (due to air trapping), usually with varying degrees of peribronchial cuffing and interstitial infiltrates. Air space shadowing may also be seen, as well as any combination of lobar collapse and consolidation.
- Radiographic resolution may lag behind clinical resolution by 2–3 weeks.

CLINICAL HOT LIST

- It is the commonest lower respiratory tract infection in infancy. Peak incidence is at 3 months, and 2% require hospital admission.
- Respiratory syncitial virus (RSV) is isolated in 75%, but there are many other potential viral pathogens.
- Clinical features include: coryza, low-grade fever, cough, tachypnoea, wheeze, recession, hyperinflation and cyanosis. The disease is more severe in babies with an underlying cardiorespiratory disorder.
- Clinical differential diagnosis includes pneumonia, cardiac failure and aspiration.
- Treatment is supportive; oxygen therapy, witholding feeds, IV fluids and occasionally ventilation (1% of admissions). There is no clinically important benefit from steroids or bronchodilators.

FURTHER READING

Baumer JH. 2007: SIGN guideline on bronchiolitis in infants. *Arch Dis Child Ed Pract;* 92: ep149–51.

Bramson RT, Griscom NT, Cleveland RH. 2005: Interpretation of chest radiographs in infants with cough and fever. Radiology; 236: 22–29.

Case 48

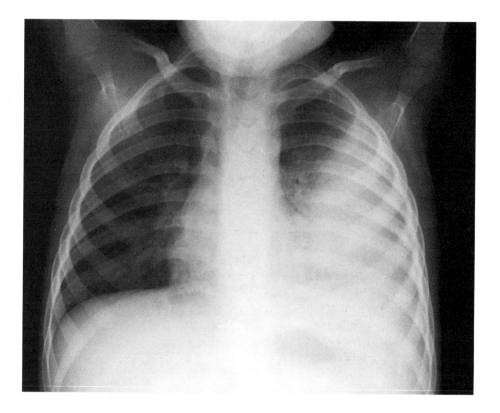

This 3-year-old boy was treated by his GP for a chest infection for 1 week. He continued to be pyrexial, and a CXR was obtained.

1. Name three abnormalities seen on the CXR.
2. What is the diagnosis?

ANSWERS

1. Within the left hemithorax there is dense opacification of the mid and lower zones that has a curved superior margin. There is loss of the clarity of the left heart border and hemidiaphragm. The trachea is deviated to the right.
2. A large left pleural empyema, with left basal consolidation.

RADIOLOGY HOT LIST

- The appearance of pleural effusions in children may differ from that in adults—fluid often parallels the chest wall, appearing as a peripheral opaque band (lamellar effusion).

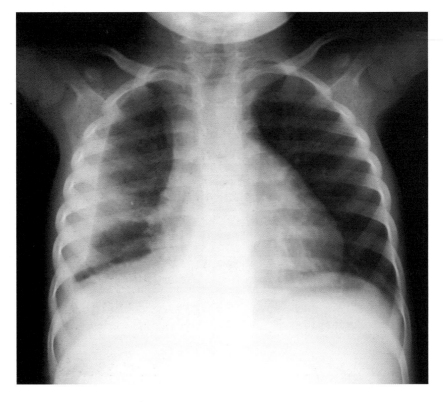

- Large pleural effusions may result in complete opacification of the hemithorax and cause tracheal deviation *away* from the side of the opaque hemithorax.
- Effusions are difficult to see on a supine film, usually producing an overall increase in density on the affected side.
- There is often an associated pneumonic process in children, so look for areas of collapse and consolidation.
- Ultrasound will confirm the presence of fluid (anechoic in simple effusions), identify loculated collection and guide percutaneous drainage.
- Contrast-enhanced CT scans will help to distinguish an empyema from a simple effusion by demonstrating enhancing pleural thickening in the former.

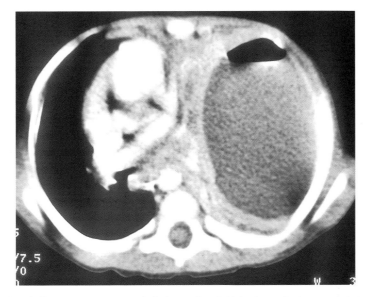

Large left pleural effusion containing gas, which shows pleural thickening and enhancement in keeping with an empyema. Note the significant mass effect, with mediastinal shift to the right.

CLINICAL HOT LIST

- Simple reactive pleural effusions often complicate bacterial pneumonia. Superadded infection results in an empyema, which may require drainage (usually percutaneous, but surgical decortication may be required for complex organized collections).
- Causes of childhood pleural effusions are:

Type of effusion	Causes
Transudate (protein < 30 g/l)	Cardiac failure, capillary leak due to sepsis, hepatic failure, nephrotic syndrome
Exudate (protein > 30 g/l)	Infection, malignancy, infarction, chylous effusion
Haemorrhagic	Trauma, bleeding disorders

FURTHER READING

Balfour-Lynn I, Abrahamson E, Cohen G et al. 2005: BTS guidelines for the management of pleural infection in children. *Thorax;* 60(Suppl I): i1–i21 or www.brit-thoracic.org.uk.

Calder A, Owens CM. 2009: Imaging of parapneumonic pleural effusions and empyema in children. *Pediatr Radiol;* 39: 1432–1998.

Case 49

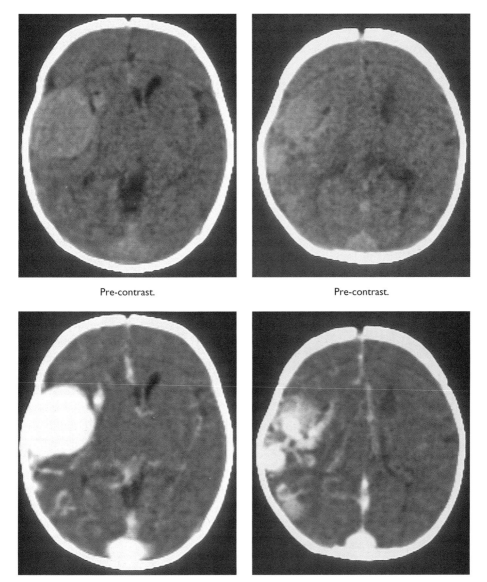

Pre-contrast.

Pre-contrast.

Post-contrast.

Post-contrast.

This 2-week-old boy presented with high-output cardiac failure.

1. What abnormalities are seen on the pre- and post-contrast CT scans of the brain?
2. What is the diagnosis?

ANSWERS

1. There is a round, well-circumscribed and hyperdense lesion in the right temporal lobe. It is causing mass effect with midline shift and effacement of the anterior horn of the right lateral ventricle. After contrast it shows intense uniform enhancement, with multiple adjacent abnormal vessels. The superior sagittal sinus shows early enhancement.
2. Right temporal arteriovenous malformation (AVM) with shunting.

RADIOLOGY HOT LIST

● Contrast-enhanced CT of an AVM will usually demonstrate dense enhancement, with large feeding vessels and draining veins. MRI will show characteristic areas of signal void in the vessels.
● A large AVM may cause obstructive hydrocephalus. Other complications include haemorrhage, infarction and local atrophy.
● A vein of Galen malformation is an AVM that arises in the midline and drains directly into an enlarged vein of Galen. It may be detected on antenatal ultrasound.
● CT or MR angiography can define the vascular anatomy prior to surgery or embolization.

CLINICAL HOT LIST

● AVMs are congenital abnormalities consisting of anomalous tortuous arteries and veins, creating an arteriovenous shunt without an intermediary capillary bed.
● Modes of presentation are:

Age group	Typical presentation
Neonatal (0–1 month)	High-output cardiac failure due to massive shunting
Infant (1–12 months)	Obstructive hydrocephalus, seizures
> 1 year	Headaches, focal neurology, hydrocephalus, haemorrhage

● Therapeutic options include embolization of arterial feeding vessels and complex neurosurgery.

FURTHER READING

Tebruegge MO, Shrivastava A. 2006: Giant cerebral arteriovenous malformation. *Arch Dis Child;* 91: 895.

Case 50

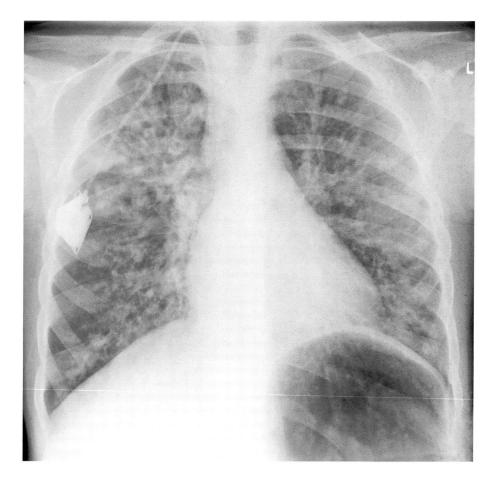

This child has been under long-term follow up for recurrent chest infections.

1. What abnormalities are seen on the chest radiograph?
2. What is the likely diagnosis?

ANSWERS

1. The lungs are hyperinflated, with widespread pulmonary infiltrates in all zones and bronchial wall thickening. There is ring shadowing due to bronchiectasis. There is a right-sided portacath in place.
2. Cystic fibrosis.

RADIOLOGY HOT LIST

- Typical features of cystic fibrosis on CXR include:

Bronchiectasis	Parallel 'tram lines', ring shadows
Peribronchial thickening	Thickened bronchial walls visible
Hyperinflation	Low, flattened diaphragms
Mucus plugging	Collapse, consolidation, air trapping
Fibrotic change	Reticular–cystic pattern of fibrosis
Hilar lymphadenopathy and/or pulmonary artery dilatation secondary to pulmonary hypertension	Prominent hila
Recurrent pneumonia	Focal areas of collapse/consolidation
Long-term intravenous access	Central venous lines, portacaths

- Be aware that in the early stages hyperinflation may be the only abnormality.
- Think of the diagnosis in a child with recurrent chest infections.

CLINICAL HOT LIST

- It is an autosomal recessive multisystem disorder and the commonest cause of chronic lung disease and exocrine pancreatic insufficiency in childhood.
- Incidence (in the UK) is 1 : 2500, heterozygotes 1 : 25.
- It is due to a gene mutation on the long arm of chromsome 7, encoding for the cystic fibrosis transmembrane conductance regulator. > 450 gene mutations have been identified, 70% ΔF508.
- Presentations include chronic respiratory symptoms, recurrent chest infections, failure to thrive, meconium ileus, malabsorption with steatorrhea, rectal prolapse and nasal polyps.
- Management strategies include diet, pancreatic supplements, physiotherapy, appropriate antibiotics, bronchodilators and DNAase.
- Survival is 75% to 18 years with good care.

FURTHER READING

Smyth RL. 2005: Diagnosis and management of cystic fibrosis. *Arch Dis Child Ed Pract;* 90: ep1–6.

Case 51

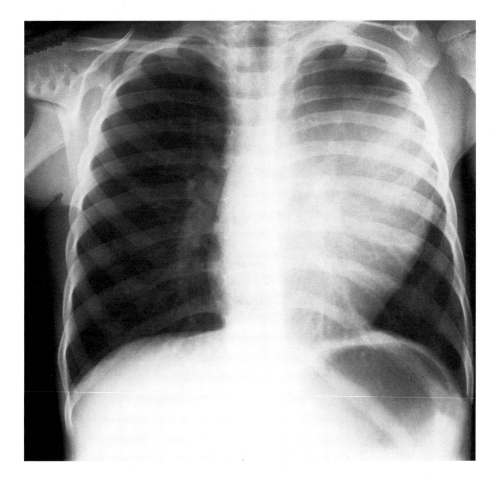

This 2-and-a-half-year-old boy presented to his GP with a 4-week history of lethargy, fever and night sweats.

1. What abnormality is seen on the CXR?
2. What is the most likely diagnosis?
3. What is the differential diagnosis?

ANSWERS

1. There is a soft tissue mass projected over the left hemithorax. The left heart border and superior mediastinal outlines are obscured, but the hilum and paraspinal line are visible through the mass. This indicates that the mass lies in the anterior mediastinum.
2. Lymphoblastic lymphoma/leukaemia.
3. Inflammatory lymphadenopathy (secondary to tuberculosis), Hodgkin's disease, germ cell tumours (GCTs) and thymic masses.

RADIOLOGY HOT LIST

- Mediastinal masses have a wide differential, and it is useful to consider them according to their anatomical location—superior, anterior, middle, or posterior mediastinum. This can often be determined on the plain X-ray, but most children will proceed to CT or MRI for further assessment.
- Leukaemia and non-Hodgkin's lymphoma (NHL) account for the majority of neoplastic anterior mediastinal masses in young children, with Hodgkin's disease and GCTs usually occurring in older children and adolescents. TB may occasionally result in large-volume mediastinal adenopathy and may mimic NHL. Neuroblastoma usually occurs in the posterior mediastinum.

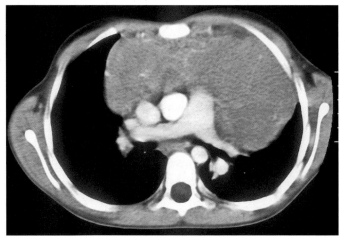

CT scan showing an anterior mediastinal mass due to lymphoma.

CLINICAL HOT LIST

- Collectively lymphoma is the third commonest childhood malignancy.
- Typically the presentation is with painless lymphadenopathy. There are usually few constitutional signs (fever, weight loss, night sweats).
- Mediastinal tumours may cause airway compromise, superior vena cava syndrome (compression of the great vessels), or oesophageal compromise.

FURTHER READING

Franco A, Mody NS, Meza MP. 2005: Imaging evaluation of pediatric mediastinal masses. *Radiol Clin N Am;* 43: 325–53.

Case 52

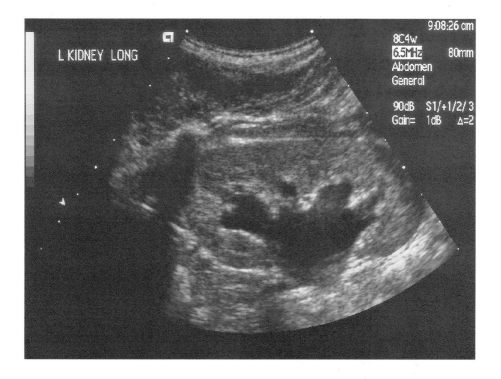

This renal ultrasound was performed on a 2-day-old girl for an antenatally detected abnormality.

1. What abnormality is seen in the left kidney?
2. What is the diagnosis?

ANSWERS

1. There is dilatation of the left pelvicalyceal system (black anechoic areas).
2. Hydronephrosis.

RADIOLOGY HOT LIST

- The calyces are only seen on ultrasound when distended by fluid.
- Ultrasound cannot reliably distinguish between the two most important causes of hydronephrosis: obstruction and vesicoureteric reflux. Further imaging studies (micturating cystourethrogram and/or nuclear medicine studies) are required to differentiate the conditions.
- If antenatal hydronephrosis is detected, postnatal investigation is recommended. Investigations include an ultrasound of the renal tract to assess renal size and morphology, and the degree of hydronephrosis. A micturating cystogram is required to exclude reflux (up to 30%), and to exclude posterior urethral valves in boys. A DMSA scan is often performed primarily to assess differential renal function and to exclude scarring. Local practice varies.
- A normal postnatal ultrasound does not exclude reflux.

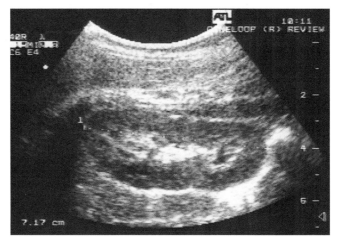

Ultrasound appearance of a normal kidney.

CLINICAL HOT LIST

- Renal pelvis dilatation is the most frequent antenatally detected abnormality (incidence 1–5%). Many of these will have no significant renal abnormality.
- More severe dilatation (> 12 mm AP pelvic diameter) may suggest obstruction (posterior urethral valves, pelvi-ureteric or vesicoureteric obstruction) or vesicoureteric reflux.
- There is currently no consensus as to follow-up imaging or the need for postnatal antibiotics.

FURTHER READING

Lee RS, Cendron M, Kinnamon DD et al. 2006: Antenatal hydronephrosis as a predictor of postnatal outcome: a meta-analysis. *Pediatrics;* 118: 586–93.

Case 53

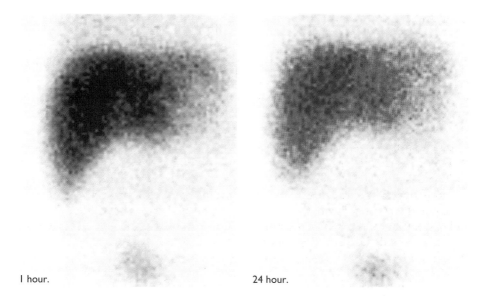

1 hour.   24 hour.

This 3-week-old boy was noted by the community midwife to have persisting jaundice. Ultrasound showed a non-dilated biliary tree but the gallbladder was not visualized. This HIDA scan (hepatic nuclear medicine scan) was carried out as part of his investigations.

1. What does it show?
2. What is the diagnosis?
3. What is the differential diagnosis for this presentation?

ANSWERS

1. The HIDA scan shows uptake of tracer by the liver, but no excretion into the small bowel. The appearance remains unchanged over 24 hours. (Normal activity is seen in the urinary bladder.)

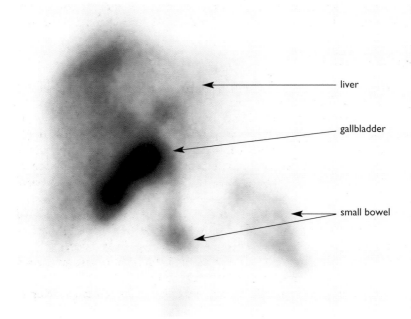

Normal HIDA scan, showing activity in the GB and small bowel at 20 minutes.

2. Biliary atresia.
3. Other causes of persisting neonatal jaundice include infectious hepatitis (toxoplasmosis, rubella and cytomegalovirus), haemolysis, metabolic abnormalities such as alpha 1 anti-trypsin deficiency, enzyme deficiencies, breast milk physiological jaundice and bile duct obstruction (inspissated bile syndrome, choledocal cyst).

RADIOLOGY HOT LIST

- Ultrasound examination is the initial radiological investigation of choice for persisting neonatal jaundice. Its main role is exclusion of a choledocal cyst or dilatation of the extrahepatic biliary system.
- HIDA scans are usually sensitive in differentiating biliary atresia from other causes of neonatal jaundice. The tracer is rapidly taken up by hepatocytes and excreted into the biliary system, gallbladder and GI tract. Visualization of tracer within the bowel indicates patency of the extrahepatic biliary system and excludes biliary atresia (with the exception of severe neonatal hepatitis or hepatic necrosis).

- Neonatal hepatitis and biliary atresia may be indistinguishable on ultrasound. The intrahepatic and extrahepatic biliary tree is typically not dilated in either condition. The gallbladder is usually absent in biliary atresia (approximately 20% of biliary atresia cases have an identifiable GB, but this is usually small). Absence of the gallbladder therefore supports a diagnosis of biliary atresia rather than neonatal hepatitis.
- Other anomalies associated with biliary atresia include preduodenal portal vein, interruption of the inferior vena cava (IVC), polysplenia (10%), and malrotation.

CLINICAL HOT LIST

- Biliary atresia is a rare congenital abnormality of unknown aetiology, incidence 1 : 15,000 live births. Biliary atresia occurs more commonly in male infants (2 : 1).
- There are two phenotypes: 90% single anomaly, 10% biliary atresia/splenic malformation syndrome (with polysplenia, situs inversus, cardiac abnormalities).
- Presentation is with prolonged jaundice with obstruction (pale stools and dark urine), failure to thrive and hepatomegaly. There is conjugated hyperbilirubinaemia. Jaundice that persists beyond 4 weeks of age is due to neonatal hepatitis or bilary atresia in 90% of cases.
- Treatment of biliary atresia is surgical, either with a portoenterostomy (Kasai procedure—only 12% cases are suitable for direct anastamotic drainage) or liver transplantation (for unsuitable cases or those with end-stage liver disease).
- Early diagnosis is therefore important as the prognosis in biliary atresia is significantly improved if surgery is performed before 10 weeks of age.
- Delay in diagnosis leads to cholestasis, fibrosis and cirrhosis (which can develop in 60 days).
- Liver biopsy may be necessary to distinguish between biliary atresia and neonatal hepatitis.
- Supportive medical management includes antibiotics, ursodeoxycholic acid, fat-soluble vitamins and attention to nutrition.

FURTHER READING

Kelly DA, Davenport M. 2007: Current management of biliary atresia. *Arch Dis Child;* 92: 1132–35.

Case 54

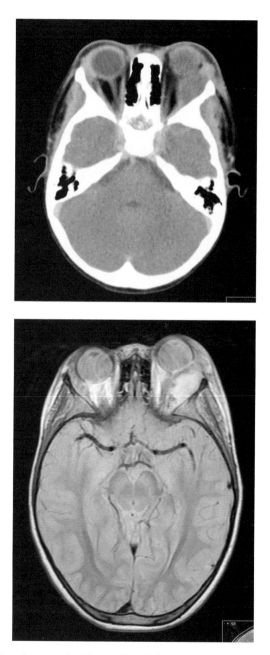

This 5-year-old boy has a painful, swollen left eye. On examination, he has a left proptosis and limited eye movements.

1. What do the CT and MRI scans of the orbits show?
2. What is the diagnosis?

ANSWERS

1. There is a left proptosis, with the globe of the left eye displaced anteromedially. This is due to an intra-orbital postseptal, extra-conal collection adjacent to the left lateral orbital wall.
2. Left orbital cellulitis with an intra-orbital abscess.

RADIOLOGY HOT LIST

- The orbital septum divides the soft tissues of the eyelid (pre-septal space) from those of the orbit (postseptal space). The extraocular muscles subdivide the postseptal space into the intraconal and extraconal spaces. The intraconal space contains the optic nerve and retrobulbar fat.
- Periorbital (pre-septal) cellulitis occurs anterior to the orbital septum and is confined to the anterior superficial orbital soft tissues. In orbital cellulitis, the infection is localized posterior to the orbital septum in the postseptal space.
- CT can distinguish between pre-septal and postseptal cellulitis and identify retro-orbital and subperiosteal collections. It may show any underlying pathology such as sinusitis.
- MRI is also useful for assessing intracranial extension of the infection into the cavernous sinus and for evaluating possible cavernous sinus thrombosis.

CLINICAL HOT LIST

- Periorbital cellulitis is a common infection of childhood and potentially serious.
- Pre-septal cellulitis represents with a superficial infection. It may result from trauma, contiguous infection or occasionally primary bacteraemia. It is commonly managed medically with antibiotics; there is a low threshold for intravenous antibiotics as posterior spread is the concern.
- Postseptal (orbital) infection is clinically more dangerous. Significant complications include visual loss (orbital involvement), cavernous sinus thrombosis, meningitis, subdural empyema and brain abscess. It may occur as a complication of acute or chronic sinusitis, or of direct spread of superficial infection. Intravenous antibiotics are required and surgical evacuation may be needed if either a subperiosteal or orbital abscess is identified.
- Clinically it may be difficult to distinguish between pre- and postseptal cellulitis, especially as this infection is frequently seen in young children. Proptosis, pain on eye movement, visual disturbance or pupilary abnormality suggests retro-orbital infection. Imaging is therefore very helpful.

FURTHER READING

Reid JR. 2004: Complications of pediatric paranasal sinusitis. *Pediatr Radiol;* 34: 933–42.

Case 55

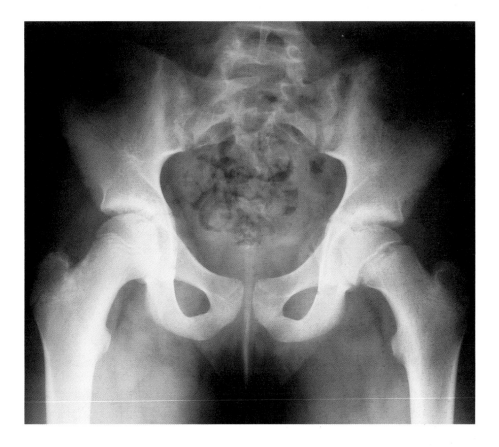

This 14-year-old girl presented to A & E with a 2-week history of a left-sided limp.

1. What is the diagnosis?

ANSWERS

1. There is a slipped femoral capital epiphysis on the left.

RADIOLOGY HOT LIST

- Epiphyseal slip may be difficult to identify on the plain AP X-ray. It is usually more obvious on the frog lateral view, which should be obtained in older children with hip pain.
- The slip is posteromedial in 99% of cases.
- Radiographic signs include:
  — widening of the epiphyseal plate.
  — reduction in the apparent height of the epiphysis.
  — a line drawn tangential to the lateral border of the femoral neck should normally pass through the lateral aspect of the femoral capital epiphysis.
  — displacement of the medial femoral metaphysis so that it no longer overlies the acetabulum.

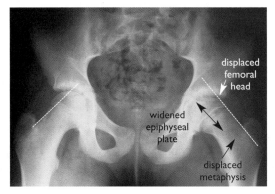

Normal hip on right and abnormal hip on left showing radiographic signs of slipped femoral epiphysis.

CLINICAL HOT LIST

- It classically occurs at the time of the pubertal growth spurt (girls aged 10–13 years, boys aged 12–15 years). There is an increased incidence in boys and overweight children (50% have weight > 95% percentile). Bilateral slip is present in 20–40% of cases.
- Symptoms include pain in the groin or knee, limp and inability to weightbear.
- There is an association with endocrine abnormalities (hypothyroidism, growth hormone treatment), radiotherapy and renal failure.
- Treatment aims to prevent further slippage with surgical pinning, and prophylactic pinning of the other hip may be required.
- Complications include avascular necrosis, acute cartilage necrosis (chondrolysis), premature physeal closure with subsequent limb-length discrepancy and premature osteoarthritis.

FURTHER READING

Hubbard AM. 2001: Imaging of pediatric hip disorders. *Radiol Clin N Am;* 39: 721–73.

Case 56

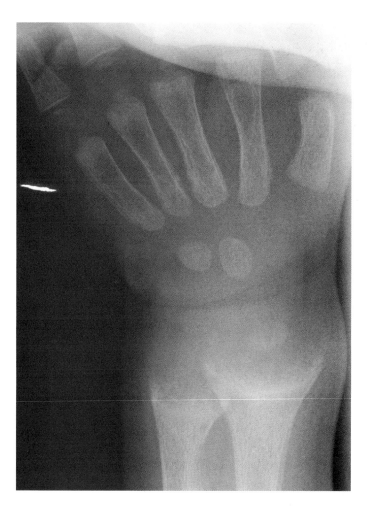

This 3-year-old child has swollen wrists.

1. What does the X-ray show?
2. What is the diagnosis?

ANSWERS

1. The bones are osteopenic. There is cupping, fraying and irregularity of the metaphyses of the distal radius and ulna.
2. Rickets.

RADIOLOGY HOT LIST

- Radiological change is seen at the distal ends of long bones, at the sites of most rapid growth: changes are most evident at the wrists and knees. There may be cupping of the anterior ribs at the costochondral junction ('rickety rosary').
- Look for leg bowing in weightbearing children, pathological fractures, generalized osteopenia and skull bossing in severe cases.
- The radiological manifestations of rickets cannot reliably distinguish between the different aetiologies.
- Rickets may be an incidental finding on the CXR—always look at the humeral metaphyses.

CLINICAL HOT LIST

- Failure of mineralization of osteoid leads to bone softening and deformity.
- Classification of rickets is as follows:

Nutritional	Dietary deficiency of vitamin D and lack of sunlight
Malabsorption	Coeliac disease, hepatobiliary disease
Hereditary renal	X-linked hypophosphataemia, vitamin D-dependent rickets, Fanconi's syndrome, distal renal tubular acidosis
Acquired renal	Chronic renal failure
Neonatal rickets	Prematurity, copper deficiency, secondary to maternal osteomalacia

FURTHER READING

Dimitri P, Bishop N. 2007: Rickets. *Paediatr Child Health;* 17: 279–87.

Case 57

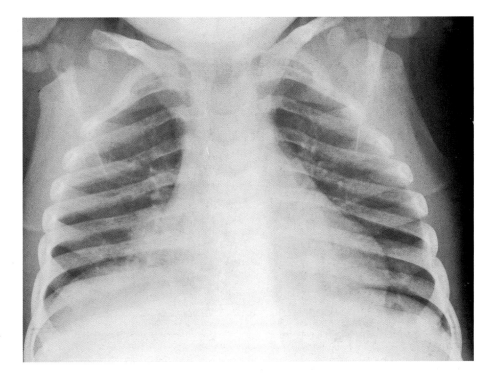

This 2-year-old boy has a cough and fever.

1. What does the CXR show?
2. What is the diagnosis?

ANSWERS

1. There is consolidation in the right mid-zone, which obscures the right heart border. The rest of the lungs are clear.
2. Right middle lobe pneumonia.

RADIOLOGY HOT LIST

- The heart borders and diaphragm are clear and distinct on a CXR as they are interfaces between radiolucent air (lung) and radio-opaque soft tissue.
- Opacification of the lung secondary to consolidation or collapse results in loss of the air–soft tissue interface—hence the ill-defined margins. The site of lung pathology can be predicted, by which the interface is obliterated:

Obscured interface	Lung lobe involved
Right heart border	Right middle lobe
Right hemidiaphragm	Right lower lobe
Right paratracheal	Right upper lobe
Left heart border	Lingula (left upper lobe)
Left hemidiaphragm	Left lower lobe

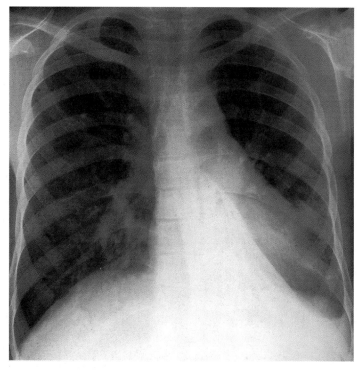

Left lower lobe collapse causing a triangular-shaped density behind the heart, and loss of the normal medial left hemidiaphragm contour.

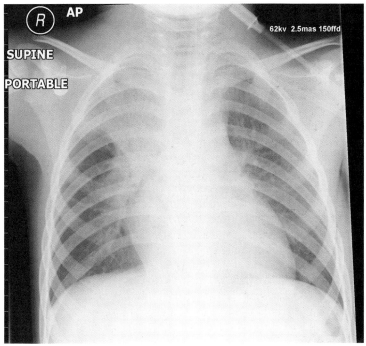

Right upper lobe collapse/consolidation with right upper zone opacification, loss of the right superior mediastinal interface and elevation of the horizontal fissure.

- Pure collapse without consolidation (such as may occur with a sputum plug or foreign body) can be very difficult to see.

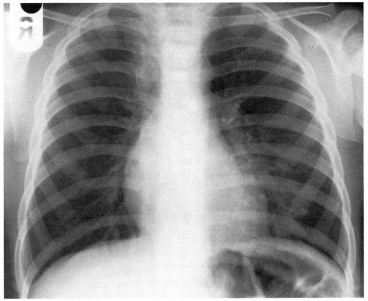

Right upper lobe collapse with widening of the right superior mediastinum, and loss of the well-defined right paratracheal stripe.

- Children may also develop round pneumonias—rounded focal areas of consolidation, which have the appearance of a mass lesion. Follow-up CXRs show resolution after antibiotic therapy.

CLINICAL HOT LIST

- Lobar consolidation is usually due to bacterial infection, with pneumococcus most commonly implicated. Haemophilus, mycoplasma and primary tuberculosis can give a similar appearance. *Klebsiella* infection classically shows 'bulging' of adjacent fissures.
- Clinical presentation and infectious agent vary with the age of the child:
  —Neonates rarely cough.
  —Systemic features may predominate in young children.
  —Viral pneumonia is most common in toddlers.
  —*Mycoplasma* is very common in the early school-age years.
  —Aspiration pneumonia is often seen in neurological impairment.
- Management will depend on the age, severity of illness and likely infectious agent. Most cases can be managed in the community.
- 3 million children die worldwide from pneumonia each year. Although most fatalities occur in developing countries, pneumonia remains a significant cause of morbidity in industrialized nations.

FURTHER READING

Bramson RT, Griscom NT, Cleveland RH. 2005: Interpretation of chest radiographs in infants with cough and fever. *Radiology;* 236: 22–29.

Case 58

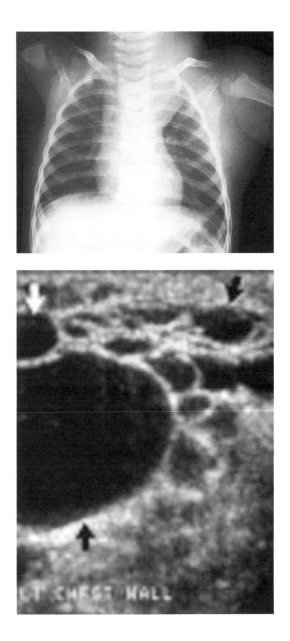

This 18-month-old girl with Turner's syndrome has a neck swelling extending into the axilla. A CXR and an USS of the swelling have been performed.

1. What does the CXR show?
2. What does the ultrasound show?
3. What is the most likely diagnosis?

ANSWERS

1. There is a large, well-circumscribed soft tissue mass on the left side of the neck, extending into the axilla and into the superior mediastinum. It displaces the trachea to the right.
2. The ultrasound shows multiple thin-walled cysts within the mass.
3. Cystic hygroma.

RADIOLOGY HOT LIST

- The mass extends from the neck into the superior mediastinum and displaces the trachea—this distinguishes it from a normal thymus gland, which does not extend above the thoracic inlet and causes no tracheal deviation.

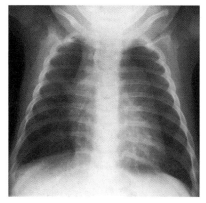

CXR showing a normal thymus.

- Ultrasound usually shows multiple thin-walled cysts.
- MRI will show a high-signal cystic mass on T2-weighted sequences, with little or no enhancement following contrast. Fluid–fluid levels are common and may indicate previous haemorrhage.

CLINICAL HOT LIST

- Cystic hygromas are macrocystic lymphatic malformations. They usually arise in the neck, and may extend into the thorax or involve the trunk. They result from maldevelopment of the cervicofacial lymphatic system.
- They are usually evident at birth and may be massive, interfering with delivery (33% incidence of perinatal demise).
- Compression of the airway, oropharynx and oesophagus is not uncommon, and may occur in smaller lesions due to sudden enlargement secondary to haemorrhage or infection. Associations include Turner's syndrome (40–80%), trisomies (13, 18, 21), Noonan's syndrome and previous exposure to teratogens (e.g. fetal alcohol syndrome).
- Treatment is usually early-staged surgical resection. Sclerosing agents can be successful.

FURTHER READING

Albanese CT, Wiener ES. 1995: Cystic hygroma. In: Spitz L, Coran AG (eds) *Pediatric Surgery*. London: Chapman & Hall, 94–99.

Koeller KK, Alamo L, Adair CF, Smirniotopoulos JG. 1999: From the Archives of the AFIP: Congenital cystic masses of the neck: Radiologic–pathologic correlation. *RadioGraphics;* 19: 121–46.

Case 59

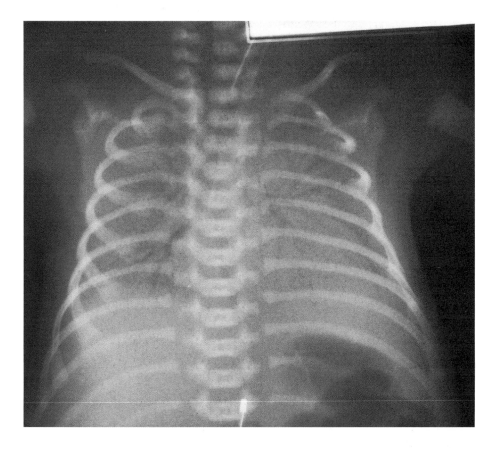

This baby was born at 26 weeks' gestation, and ventilated for respiratory distress. This CXR was taken at 36 hours.

1. Describe the CXR appearances.
2. What is the most likely diagnosis?
3. What is the differential diagnosis?

ANSWERS

1. The lungs are small volume. There is diffuse symmetrical opacification of both lungs ('ground glass'), with bilateral air bronchograms, and loss of the cardiac outline and hemidiaphragms. There is an endotracheal tube in situ.
2. Surfactant deficiency disease or hyaline membrane disease (HMD).
3. Neonatal pneumonia, pulmonary oedema and pulmonary haemorrhage.

RADIOLOGY HOT LIST

- The CXR may be normal initially. It may progress from fine reticular shadowing to complete white-out with air bronchograms and loss of the cardiac and diaphragmatic contours.
- The routine administration of surfactant and perinatal steroids means that the classic severe appearances of HMD are no longer commonly seen. Radiological findings are therefore very variable, and pulmonary infiltrates are often asymmetric.

CLINICAL HOT LIST

- Surfactant deficiency disease is synonymous with HMD and respiratory distress syndrome. Lack of surfactant causes diffuse alveolar collapse.
- It is common under 30 weeks' gestation and almost inevitable under 28 weeks.
- Other associations include asphyxia, hypothermia, haemolytic disease of the newborn and maternal diabetes.
- The incidence can be reduced by prevention of premature delivery and antenatal maternal steroids.
- Neonatal pneumonia may have an indistinguishable appearance from HMD, and antibiotic cover is required until the results of blood cultures are known.

FURTHER READING

Agrons GA, Courtney SE, Stocker JT, Markowitz RI. 2005: From the Archives of the AFIP: Lung disease in premature neonates: Radiologic-pathologic correlation. *RadioGraphics;* 25: 1047–73.

Case 60

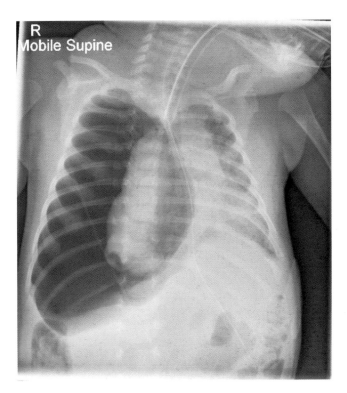

This 5-day-old baby, born at 28 weeks' gestation and ventilated for surfactant deficiency disease or hyaline membrane disease (HMD), had a sudden increase in oxygen and ventilatory requirements.

1. What abnormality is seen on the chest radiograph?
2. What is the diagnosis?

ANSWERS

1. There is a right-sided tension pneumothorax with mediastinal shift and depression of the diaphragm. There is collapse of the underlying lung.
2. Neonatal tension pneumothorax complicating hyaline membrane disease.

RADIOLOGY HOT LIST

- Neonatal pneumothorax may not have the classic appearances seen in ambulant children because the film is taken with the baby supine.
- The lung is usually displaced posteriorly in the supine patient, with free pleural air collecting anteriorly and medially. Thus the AP film may only show increased radiolucency over the entire hemithorax, or a sharp outline to the adjacent mediastinum or heart. A lung edge may not be seen.
- There may be a subpulmonary collection of air.
- If the underlying lung is stiff (e.g. from HMD) it may not collapse completely.
- Signs of a tension pneumothorax include shift of the trachea, flattening or distortion of the hemidiaphragm and mediastinal displacement.
- Pneumothorax may be associated with pneumomediastinum (air within the mediastinal space) and surgical emphysema (subcutaneous air).

CLINICAL HOT LIST

- 1–2% of all neonates will have a spontaneous pneumothorax—only half of these are symptomatic.
- Pneumothorax in the neonatal period may be secondary to mechanical ventilation, severe HMD, pulmonary interstitial emphysema and meconium aspiration.
- The incidence of iatrogenic pneumothorax in ventilated babies is decreasing as a result of surfactant and improved ventilatory strategies.
- Management depends on clinical severity; the vast majority of ventilated neonates will require a chest drain.

FURTHER READING

Donn SM, Sinha SK. 2006: Minimising ventilator induced lung injury in preterm infants. *Arch Dis Child Fetal Neonatal Ed;* 91: F226–30.

Case 61

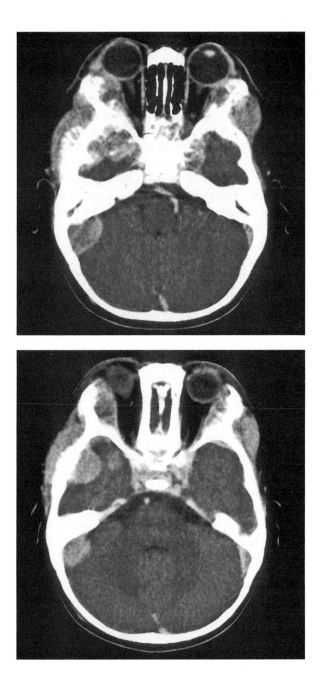

This 1-year-old boy presented with proptosis, hypertension and an abdominal mass.

1. What does the contrast-enhanced CT scan show?
2. What is the most likely diagnosis?

ANSWERS

1. There are enhancing, extracerebral, bone-based masses arising from the lateral orbital walls and the middle and posterior cranial fossae, associated with a spiculated periosteal reaction. There is bilateral proptosis.
2. Metastatic bony, peri-orbital and parameningeal neuroblastoma.

RADIOLOGY HOT LIST

- The majority of infants and children with neuroblastoma have metastases at diagnosis. They usually involve the long bones and orbits (classically the lateral wall).
- Parameningeal deposits are less common, and are secondary to haematogenous spread to the epidural space.
- Rhabdomyosarcoma may also affect the orbit, but is usually unilateral and there may be extensive local bone destruction.

CLINICAL HOT LIST

- Neuroblastoma is the most common extracranial solid malignant tumour in children.
- Neuroblastoma is usually clinically silent until it causes mass effect, invades or compresses neighbouring structures, or metastasizes. There is a wide range of clinical presentations and tumour behaviours.
- 70% of patients have disseminated disease at diagnosis, and presenting symptoms are secondary to metastatic spread or a paraneoplastic syndrome. Proptosis and bone pain are well-recognized clinical presentations. The commonest presentation is with an abdominal mass.

FURTHER READING

Chung EM, Murphey MD, Specht CS, Cube R, Smirniotopoulos J. 2008: From the Archives of the AFIP: Pediatric orbit tumors and tumorlike lesions: Osseous lesions of the orbit. *RadioGraphics;* 28: 1193–214.

Case 62

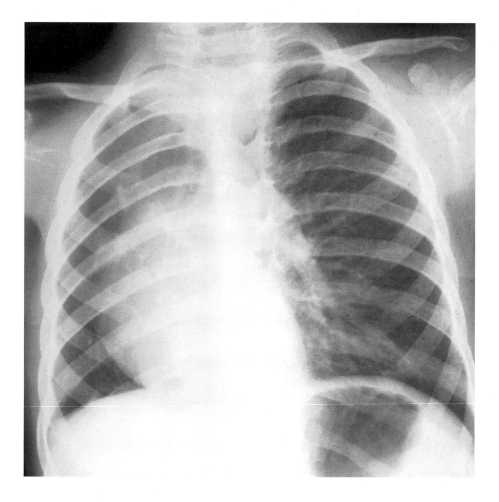

This 4-year-old boy is asymptomatic.

1. What does the CXR show?
2. What is the diagnosis?

ANSWERS

1. The right hemithorax is reduced in volume and there is mediastinal shift to this side. The right lung has reduced vascularity (right main pulmonary artery not seen and paucity of vessels peripherally). There are no focal areas of collapse or consolidation.
2. Right pulmonary hypoplasia.

RADIOLOGY HOT LIST

- Common causes of mediastinal shift include:

Towards affected side	Collapse secondary to an inhaled foreign body, mucous plug or infection. Pulmonary hypoplasia
Away from affected side	Air trapping due to an inhaled foreign body, tension pneumothorax, large pleural effusion, intrathoracic mass

- Always assess the pulmonary vasculature. The oligaemic side is usually the abnormal side!
- The small hemithorax and mediastinal shift, coupled with the diminished vascularity, indicate chronic pathology, rather than an acute pulmonary collapse. Always compare with old films.

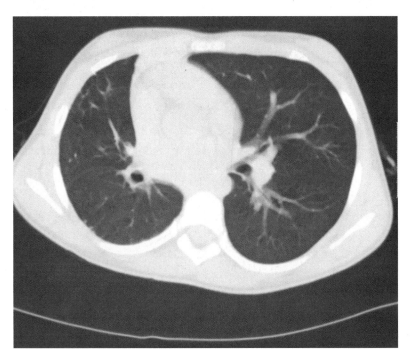

CT confirms a smaller right lung, with small pulmonary vessels and no distinct basal right basal pulmonary artery. The left lung is normal.

CLINICAL HOT LIST

- Congenital underdevelopment of one or more lobes of the lung can be differentiated into three forms:

Pulmonary agenesis	Absence of lobe and bronchus
Pulmonary aplasia	Rudimentary bronchus with no parenchyma or vessels
Pulmonary hypoplasia	Bronchus completely formed, but small. Small vessels and rudimentary parenchyma

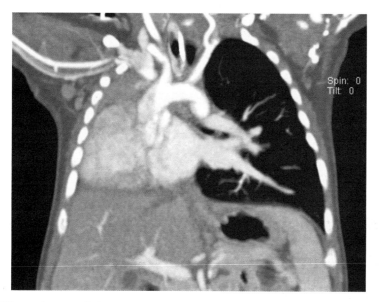

Coronal CT scan showing right lung agenesis, with the heart and mediastinum within the right hemithorax and no visible right lung.

- Idiopathic pulmonary hypoplasia is often asymptomatic and an incidental finding on CXRs. Patients may be prone to exertional dyspnoea.
- There are many causes of secondary pulmonary underdevelopment:

Small fetal thorax	Congenital diaphragmatic hernia, pleural effusion with hydrops, thoracic malformation, abdominal mass
Oligohydramnios	Fetal renal disease, premature rupture of membranes
Decreased fetal breathing	CNS abnormality, neuromuscular disease

FURTHER READING

Paterson A. 2005: Imaging evaluation of congenital lung abnormalities in infants and children. *Radiol Clin N Am;* 43: 303–23.

Case 63

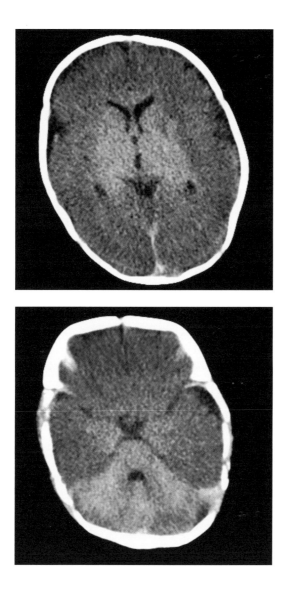

This term infant was born after emergency Caesarean section for a placental abruption. At delivery, he was white, floppy and had profound bradycardia. He was resuscitated, but has had frequent seizures since his admission to the neonatal unit. This scan was taken 48 hours after birth.

1. What does the CT brain scan show?
2. What is the diagnosis?

ANSWERS

1. There is diffuse low density in both cerebral hemispheres with loss of the normal grey–white matter differentiation (due to global cerebral ischaemia and oedema). The cerebellum, basal ganglia and thalamus appear relatively high density—the 'acute reversal sign'.
2. Hypoxic ischaemic encephalopathy (HIE).

RADIOLOGY HOT LIST

- Severe HIE may manifest as the 'acute reversal sign' on CT. This occurs due to relative preservation of cerebral perfusion to the brainstem, cerebellum and basal ganglia after the hypoxic insult.
- These features may occur after any cause of hypoxic–ischaemic insult, including NAI.
- The acute reversal sign on CT indicates an extremely poor prognosis and survivors usually have severe neurological deficit.
- MRI in the first 1–4 weeks after birth is the most accurate means of understanding the pattern and timing of injury.

CLINICAL HOT LIST

- HIE may occur after any hypoxic–ischaemic insult.
- The commonest cause of HIE is perinatal hypoxia/ischaemia. Other causes include abnormalities of metabolism and of brain development.
- The clinical picture ranges from transient irritability and poor feeding, to hypertonia and prolonged seizures.
- Outcomes range from neurological normality or subtle behavioural changes through to cerebral palsy and death.
- Early prediction of neurological outcome may be assessed by cerebral function monitoring (CFM) or an electroencephalogram (EEG). Early cranial ultrasound may show diagnoses other than HIE, cerebral injury established before birth and the evolution of acute cerebral damage.
- A standardized neurological examination 2–3 weeks after birth and observations of the quality of general movements are good bedside predictors of outcome.
- Management is largely supportive. However hypothermia within 6 hours of birth has shown modest improvements in outcome in moderately affected babies.

FURTHER READING

Chao CP, Zaleski CG, Patton AC. 2006: Neonatal hypoxic–ischemic encephalopathy: Multimodality imaging findings. *RadioGraphics;* 26: S159–72.
Cowan F, Azzopardi D. 2007: Hypoxic ischaemic encephalopathy. *Paediatr Child Health;* 17: 47–57.

Case 64

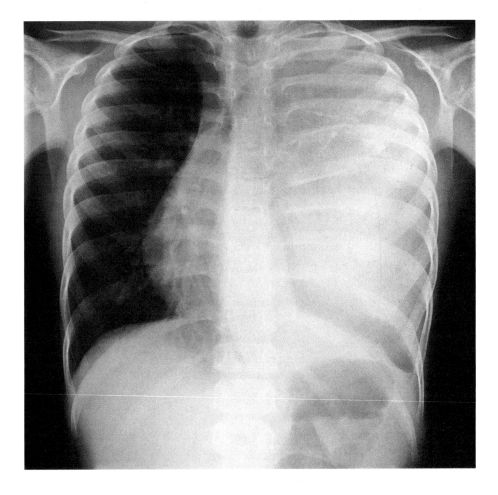

This 5-year-old girl has become increasingly short of breath and tired.

1. What does the CXR show?
2. What is the diagnosis?

ANSWERS

1. The left hemithorax is radiopaque and small areas of calcification are seen within it. There is loss of the left heart border and mediastinal shift to the right. The posterior ribs are splayed and eroded, indicating the presence of an aggressive mass lesion.
2. Thoracic neuroblastoma.

RADIOLOGY HOT LIST

- Neurogenic tumours account for 95% of posterior mediastinal masses in children.
- Look for calcification (present in 25% of thoracic neuroblastomas) and associated vertebral or rib erosion.
- Other thoracic tumours that may involve the chest wall include Ewing's sarcoma, primitive neuroectodermal tumours, rhabdomyosarcoma and lymphoma. Rhabdomyosarcoma and lymphoma do not usually calcify and bone destruction is unusual.
- MRI or CT is required to assess anatomical location and local spread, particularly paraspinal and extradural extension (extension into the spinal canal) and involvement of major vessels or trachea.

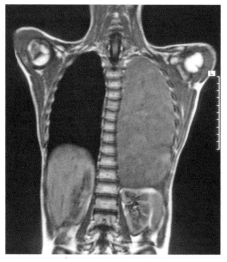

Coronal T1-weighted MRI through the patient's thorax.

CLINICAL HOT LIST

- 15% of neuroblastomas occur in the thorax, arising from the sympathetic ganglia.
- Neuroblastoma is often clinically silent until it invades or compresses adjacent structures, such as the trachea, oesophagus or spinal canal.
- Extradural spread may cause spinal cord compression with paraplegia, Horner's syndrome, or alteration in bladder or bowel function.
- Thoracic neuroblastoma has a significantly better prognosis than abdominal neuroblastoma, probably due to earlier clinical presentation.

FURTHER READING

Hildebrandt T, Traunecker H. 2005: Neuroblastoma: A tumour with many faces. *Curr Paed;* 15: 412–20.

Case 65

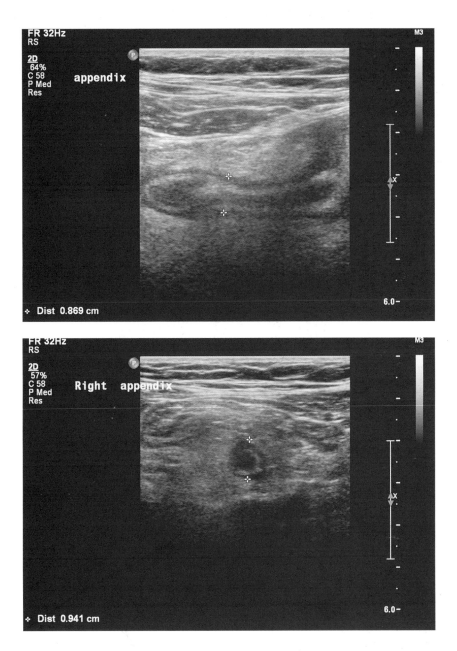

This 12-year-old boy was admitted via A & E with fever, abdominal pain and vomiting.

1. What abnormality is shown on the ultrasound image of the right iliac fossa?
2. What is the diagnosis?

ANSWERS

1. There is a tubular, blind-ending and thick-walled loop of bowel in the right iliac fossa, in keeping with the appendix. There is increased echogenicity of the surrounding fat, suggesting inflammation.
2. Acute appendicitis.

RADIOLOGY HOT LIST

● Ultrasound is the first-line investigation for appendicitis in children and young adults. Ultrasound may be diagnostic and may demonstrate any of the following: a typical tubular structure with a cross-section diameter > 6 mm, a complex mass, appendicolith, evidence of inflammatory change in the peri-appendiceal fat, free fluid.

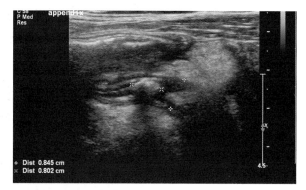

There is an appendicolith with posterior shadowing within the proximal inflamed appendix.

● An appendix abscess may be detected as a soft tissue mass or complex fluid collection.
● The plain AXR is usually normal, but an appendicolith may be visible (> 90% probability of appendicitis in a child with abdominal pain). There may be small bowel dilatation secondary to an ileus or small bowel obstruction.
● The diagnosis is not excluded by negative ultrasound imaging. CT (which carries a significant radiation burden) should be reserved for equivocal cases, and is usually diagnostic.

CLINICAL HOT LIST

● Appendicitis is the commonest surgical emergency of childhood (incidence 4 : 1000).
● Symptoms in older children are similar to those seen in adults. The cardinal sign is tenderness at McBurney's point. In younger children presentation may be with anorexia, fever, irritability, diarrhoea and vomiting. The incidence of perforation is higher in younger children.
● The differential diagnosis includes non-specific abdominal pain, gastroenteritis, mesenteric adenitis, Henoch–Schönlein purpura, constipation, urinary tract infection, lower lobe pneumonia and diabetes.
● Treatment consists of resuscitation and appendicectomy. An appendix mass may be managed conservatively.

FURTHER READING

Birnbaum BA, Wilson SR. 2000: Appendicitis at the millennium. *Radiology;* 215: 337–48.

Case 66

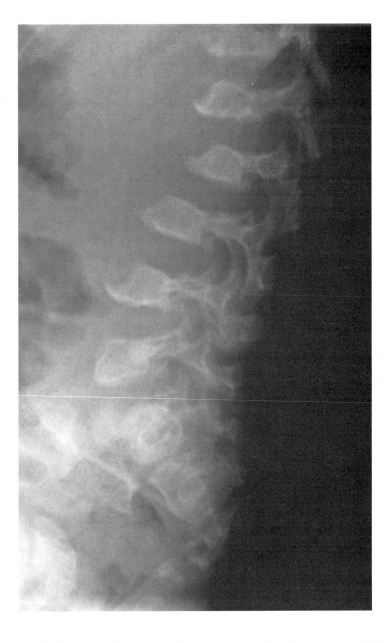

This 2-year-old boy is under investigation for progressive developmental delay. On examination he is short, has coarse facial features and hepatosplenomegaly.

1. What does the lateral X-ray of the lumbar spine show?
2. What is the most likely diagnosis?
3. What is the differential diagnosis?

ANSWERS

1. There is a mild kyphosis at the thoracolumbar junction. The vertebral bodies are abnormal with anterior inferior beaking and long slender pedicles.
2. Mucopolysaccharidosis: Hurler's syndrome.
3. Other causes of anterior inferior beaking of the vertebral bodies include achondroplasia and hypothyroidism.

RADIOLOGY HOT LIST

● Skeletal dysplasia is a component of Hurler's syndrome, with widespread radiographic abnormalities involving the axial skeleton and extremities.
● The earliest radiographic changes involve the skull: frontal bossing, calvarial thickening and a J-shaped sella. The characteristic features in the spine are described above. The iliac bones are flared. The ribs are 'oar shaped'.
● The hands are abnormal ('trident hands'): broad expanded metacarpals with tapered proximal ends.

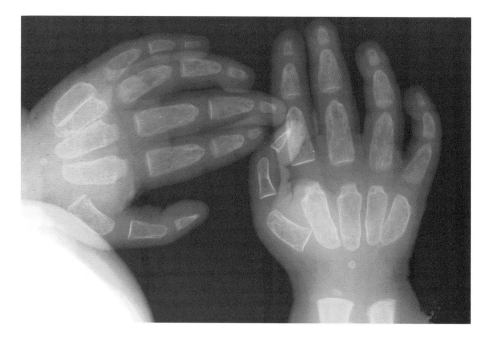

CLINICAL HOT LIST

● The mucopolysaccharidoses are a complex heterogeneous group of lysosomal storage disorders, with abnormalities of mucopolysaccharide or glycoprotein metabolism.
● Classification depends on the particular enzyme deficiency. There are seven types in total. Babies are usually normal at birth, but develop multisystem disease by 2 years. Neurological and developmental regression will depend on subtype.

MPS II (Hunter's syndrome) is X linked; the others are autosomal recessive:

Type	Inheritance	Neurological signs	Somatic features	Prognosis
I–Hurler	Autosomal recessive	Marked retardation	Coarse facies, short stature, skeletal dysplasia, corneal clouding, hepato-splenomegaly, valvular heart disease	Death in childhood, bone marrow transplant curative
II–Hunter	X-linked	Mild retardation	As for Hurler's (but no corneal clouding)	Survive to adulthood
IV–Morquio	Autosomal dominant	Normal	Normal face, short stature, marked kyphosis, hypotonia, contractures	Survive to adulthood

FURTHER READING

Wraith JE. 1995: The mucopolysaccharidoses: a clinical review and guide to management *Arch Dis Child;* 72: 263–7.

Case 67

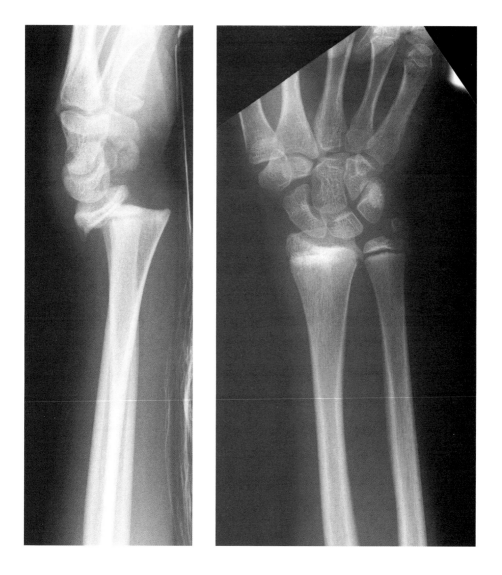

A 13-year-old boy was brought to casualty following an injury on the football pitch.

1. What abnormality is demonstrated on the plain radiograph?
2. What is the diagnosis?
3. What is the significance of recognizing this injury?

ANSWERS

1. There is posterior displacement of the distal radial epiphysis, which is only appreciated on the lateral view. This illustrates the importance of two views at right angles when assessing trauma.
2. A Salter–Harris type I epiphyseal injury.
3. Epiphyseal fractures may require open reduction to avoid angulation and/or premature fusion with consequent limb shortening.

RADIOLOGY HOT LIST

- The epiphyseal complex (epiphysis, cartilagenous growth plate, and metaphysis) is involved in 6–15% of paediatric fractures, most commonly at the wrist and the ankle.
- It is important to recognize fractures involving the growth plate as orthopaedic intervention may be required.

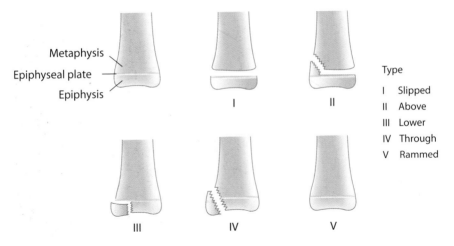

SALTR – This is a useful mnemonic, describing the relation of the fracture to the epiphyseal plate.

- Complex fractures may require preoperative CT to assess the position of bony fragments and aid surgical planning. 3D volume-rendered CT images allow better spatial appreciation of complex fractures.

CLINICAL HOT LIST

- Types I, II and III fractures are treated by closed reduction and immobilization.
- Types IV and V fractures require open reduction and internal fixation to prevent premature growth plate fusion with subsequent limb shortening and angulation.

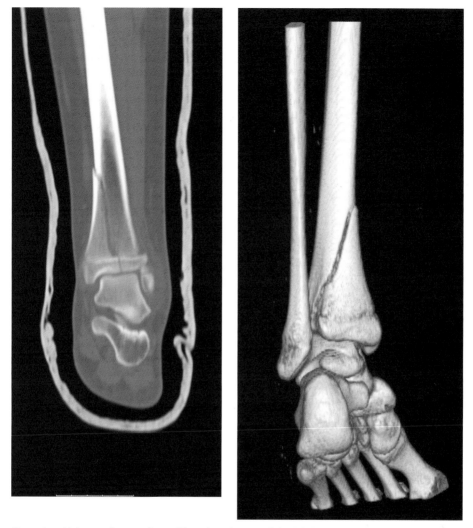

Coronal multiplanar reformat of type IV epiphyseal injury of the left distal tibia, with a volume-rendered reformat of the same fracture.

Case 68

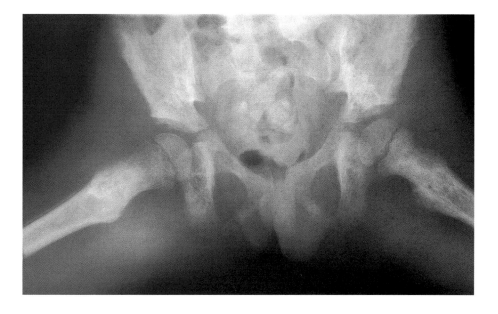

This 5-year-old boy presented with right-sided hip pain and bruising. The full blood count showed anaemia and thrombocytopaenia, but a high white cell count.

1. Comment on the X-ray of the pelvis.
2. What is the likely diagnosis?

ANSWERS

1. The bone texture is diffusely abnormal throughout, with a permeative, moth-eaten appearance. There are bilateral symmetrical periosteal reactions along both femoral shafts.
2. Acute lymphoblastic leukaemia.

RADIOLOGY HOT LIST

- Skeletal manifestations occur in 50–90% of leukaemia patients and are usually due to leukaemic infiltration. X-ray changes may precede blood film abnormalities, and resolve with successful therapy.
- The appearances may include osteoporosis, transverse lucent metaphyseal bands, focal osteolytic lesions and periosteal reactions.
- Similar radiological features are seen with metastatic neuroblastoma.

CLINICAL HOT LIST

Pathology	Clinical manifestation
Bone marrow failure	Anaemia, thrombocytopaenia, neutropenia
Tissue and organ infiltration	Splenomegaly, lymphadenopathy, bone involvement
Systemic effects	Fever, lethargy, anorexia

- Treatment includes:
1. Chemotherapy (remission of induction then maintenance).
2. Radiotherapy.
3. Bone marrow transplantation (BMT).
4. Supportive measures (blood transfusions and prevention/treatment of infection).

FURTHER READING

Chessells JM. 2000: Recent advances in management of acute leukaemia. *Arch Dis Childhood;* 82: 438–42.

Sinigaglia R, Gigante C, Bisivella G et al. 2008: Musculoskeletal manifestation in paediatric leukaemia. *J Pediatr Orthop;* 28: 20–8.

Case 69

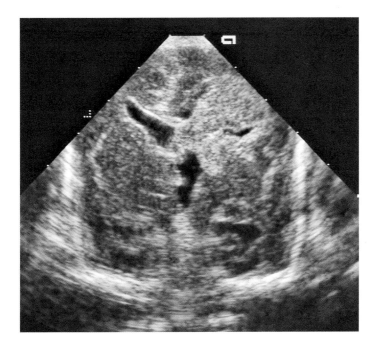

This 3-day-old baby was born at 27 weeks' gestation and ventilated for severe hyaline membrane disease. He suddenly collapsed on the ventilator with hypotension, metabolic acidosis and hypotonia. A cranial USS was performed.

1. What abnormality is seen?
2. What are the possible sequelae to this?

ANSWERS

1. There is a mass of increased echogenicity seen within the left lateral ventricle and periventricular white matter of the left frontal lobe. This represents a grade IV intraventricular haemorrhage with parenchymal extension. There is dilatation of the left temporal horn secondary to the obstructing clot.
2. Intraventricular haemorrhage may cause death. In those infants who survive, there may be hydrocephalus and periventricular leukomalacia, with long-term neurological disability.

RADIOLOGY HOT LIST

- The blood clot appears as an amorphous mass of high echogenicity that may fill the ventricle, or layer in the dependent part of the ventricle.
- Assess ventricular dilatation, and the adjoining cerebral parenchyma for periventricular involvement.
- On parasagittal scans, the echogenic choroid plexus does not extend beyond the caudothalamic groove, so any high echogenicity seen in the anterior horns of the lateral ventricles is pathological.
- Classification is as follows:

Grade 1	Confined to subependymal germinal matrix
Grade 2	Extension into non-dilated ventricles
Grade 3	Extension into dilated ventricles
Grade 4	Massive intraventricular and intraparenchymal haemorrhage

CLINICAL HOT LIST

- Haemorrhage occurs in the germinal layer (vascular network, floor of lateral ventricles). This normally involutes in the later part of pregnancy, and thus periventricular haemorrhage (PVH) is not usually seen in infants over 32 weeks' gestation.
- It affects 20% of neonates with a birthweight below 1.5 kg.
- It is commonly asymptomatic, particularly grades 1 and 2, and therefore routine scanning is necessary on neonatal intensive care units.
- Risk factors include hypotension, hypoxia, acidosis, respiratory distress syndrome and pneumothorax.
- Grades 1 and 2 have a good prognosis. Virtually all those with grade 4 lesions will have neurological impairment.

FURTHER READING

Levene M. 2005: The sequelae of periventricular haemorrhage. *Curr Paed;* 15: 375–80.

Case 70

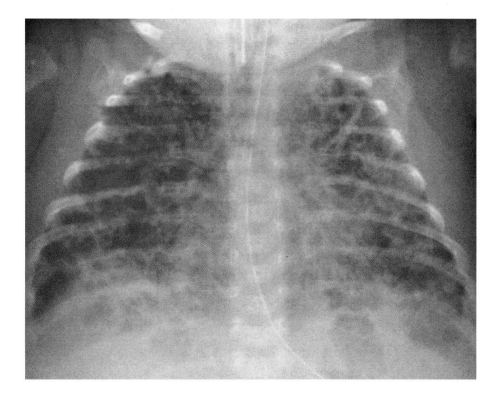

This 5-week-old baby was born at 26 weeks' gestation and has been ventilated since birth.

1. What abnormalities are seen on the CXR?
2. What is the diagnosis?

206

ANSWERS

1. The lungs are hyperinflated. There is coarse reticular shadowing with rounded lucent areas in both lungs. The heart and diaphragmatic outlines are ill defined.
2. Bronchopulmonary dysplasia (also known as chronic lung disease).

RADIOLOGY HOT LIST

- Bronchopulmonary dysplasia is a chronic lung disorder, and is defined as oxygen dependency after 28 days. However, the radiological changes develop during this period, usually following ventilation for hyaline membrane disease (HMD).
- The radiographic changes of BPD have been described in four stages, however the radiological features can be complex and variable and clearly defined stages are rarely seen in clinical practice.

Stage	Time	CXR appearance
I	First week	HMD
II	Second week	Generalized haziness and plethora
III	Third week	Cystic changes and stranding
IV	Fourth week	Hyperinflation, extensive stranding and emphysematous changes

- There may be complete radiological resolution over months or even years. Others may have retained linear densities and upper lobe emphysema.

CLINICAL HOT LIST

- Chronic lung disease/bronchopulmonary dysplasia is seen following ventilation of the premature neonate, and affects up to 50% of neonates with a birthweight < 750 g. There is an increased incidence due to improved survival of very low birthweight infants.
- Aetiological factors include lung immaturity, barotrauma, oxygen toxicity, infection, inflammation, patent ductus arteriosus, fluid overload, pulmonary interstitial emphysema and persistently abnormal surfactant. These lead to abnormal repair with fibroproliferative regeneration.
- Management is largely supportive, e.g. prevention of further lung injury and attention to nutrition. There is controversy about the use of steroids—they may facilitate weaning from the ventilator, but they are associated with poorer long-term neurodevelopmental outcome and cerebral palsy.

FURTHER READING

Agrons GA, Courtney SE, Stocker JT, Markowitz RI. 2005: From the Archives of the AFIP: Lung disease in premature neonates: Radiologic–pathologic correlation. *RadioGraphics;* 25: 1047–73.

Bhakta KY, Stark AR. 2006: Management of chronic lung disease of the premature infant. *Curr Paed;* 16: 165–71.

Case 71

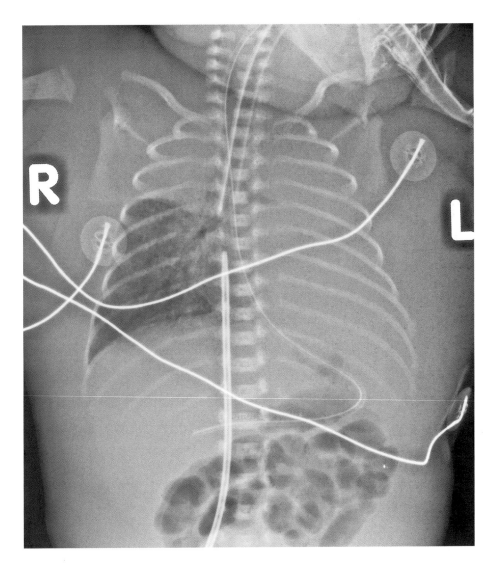

This 1-week-old baby, born at 28 weeks' gestation, is being ventilated. His oxygen requirement has increased since re-intubation, and a repeat CXR was requested.

1. What abnormalities are seen on the CXR?
2. What is the appropriate next step?

ANSWERS

1. The tip of the endotracheal tube (ETT) lies too low, in the right main bronchus. This has resulted in collapse/consolidation of the entire left lung and right upper lobe. Only the right middle and lower lobe are aerated. (Note also the oedematous soft tissues due to fluid overload.)
2. The tube should be pulled back into a more satisfactory position.

RADIOLOGY HOT LIST

- The ETT may be inserted too far at intubation. The correct position for the ETT tip is halfway between the thoracic inlet and the carina (ideally at T1).
- Flexion of the baby's neck may cause a low-lying tube to slip into the right main bronchus. The right upper lobe bronchus may be occluded by the ETT (if the tip lies in the bronchus intermedius) causing collapse/consolidation of the right upper lobe.

CLINICAL HOT LIST

- Beware! Absent chest movement may indicate an oesophageal intubation. Asymmetrical chest movement and breath sounds should raise the suspicion of a malpositioned ETT.
- Always obtain a CXR post intubation!

FURTHER READING

Wyllie JP. 2008: Neonatal endotracheal intubation. *Arch Dis Child Ed Pract*; 93: 44–9.

Case 72

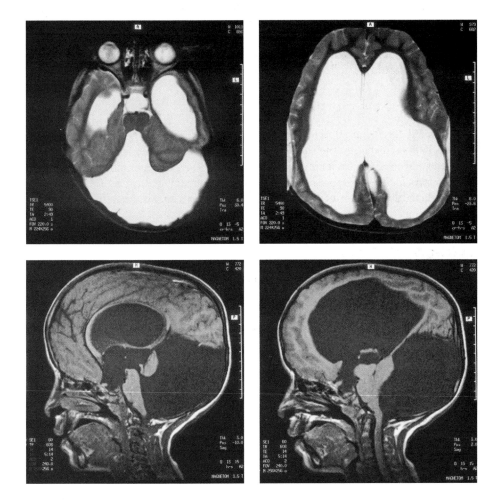

This 6-year-old child was referred for assessment from abroad. He has a large head, mild developmental delay and convulsions dating from infancy. MRI T1-weighted sagittal and T2-weighted axial images have been obtained.

1. What abnormality is demonstrated?
2. What is the diagnosis?

ANSWERS

1. There is cystic dilatation of the IVth ventricle, which fills the entire posterior fossa. There is agenesis of the cerebellar vermis, and elevation of the tentorium cerebelli. There is associated hydrocephalus.
2. Dandy–Walker malformation.

RADIOLOGY HOT LIST

- It is characterized by the absence/hypoplasia of the cerebellar vermis, and associated cerebellar hypoplasia.
- The IVth ventricle is grossly dilated, and the ensuing large posterior fossa cyst causes elevation of the tentorium.
- Hydrocephalus occurs secondary to atresia of the IVth ventricle foramina, aqueductal stenosis, or compression of the aqueduct by the cyst.
- It may be associated with other CNS abnormalities, including agenesis of the corpus callosum (seen in 25%).

CLINICAL HOT LIST

- Most cases are diagnosed on antenatal ultrasound. The child may present later (uncommon in the UK) with a large head, developmental delay, ataxia and seizures.
- 50% have learning difficulties.
- It is usually sporadic, but occasionally it is associated with abnormalities of chromosome 9.
- It may be associated with other CNS malformations and midline facial and palate defects.
- Hydrocephalus may require ventriculo-peritoneal shunting.

FURTHER READING

Epelman M, Daneman A, Blaser SI et al. 2006: Differential diagnosis of intracranial cystic lesions at head US: Correlation with CT and MR imaging. *RadioGraphics;* 26: 173–96.

Mohanty A, Biswas A, Satish S, Praharaj SS, Sastry KV. 2006: Treatment options for Dandy–Walker malformation. *J Neurosurg;* 105(5 Suppl): 348–56.

Case 73

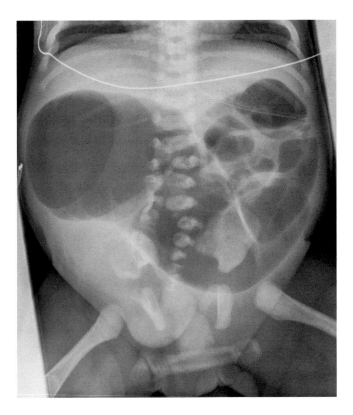

This 2-day-old baby has abdominal distension and has not passed meconium. On examination, he is found to have an imperforate anus.

1. What does the AXR show?
2. What is the underlying diagnosis?

212

ANSWERS

1. There are multiple loops of distended bowel indicating low bowel obstruction due to the underlying anorectal atresia. There are multiple lumbar vertebral abnormalities and the right side of the sacrum is hypoplastic.
2. Vertebral abnormalities in the presence of anorectal atresia are suggestive of the VATER association. The child had only one kidney.

RADIOLOGY HOT LIST

- The spine should be carefully assessed on chest and abdominal radiographs.
- The VATER association should be suspected in any child with a vertebral anomaly. At a minimum a renal USS should be performed.

CLINICAL HOT LIST

- An association is a combination of congenital abnormalities that occur together at a greater frequency than by chance alone. (A syndrome is a recognized pattern of clinical abnormalities with a single cause.)
- **VATER** = **V**ertebral abnormalities, **A**nal atresia, **T**racheo**E**sophageal fistula, **R**enal or **R**adial abnormalities
- These abnormalities are likely to be due to an insult at a specific stage of embryogenesis with effects in all these different systems.
- If one of the abnormalities detailed above is found, the others should be sought.

Case 74

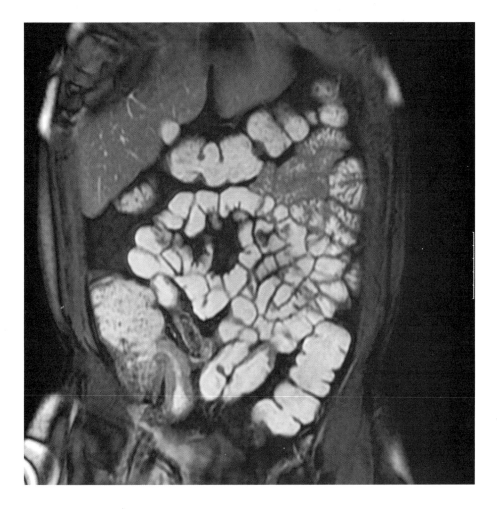

This 12-year-old boy suffers from weight loss, abdominal pain and diarrhoea.

1. What investigation has been performed?
2. What is the main abnormality?
3. What is the most likely diagnosis?

ANSWERS

1. An MRI small bowel study, with high signal fluid in the small bowel, caecum and colon.
2. The terminal ileum is abnormal, with a narrowed lumen and thickening of the bowel wall. The caecal pole is also thick walled.
3. A terminal ileal stricture secondary to Crohn's disease.

RADIOLOGY HOT LIST

- Crohn's disease affects the small bowel in 80% of cases and the terminal ileum is the commonest site of disease.
- MRI is the investigation of choice in the assessment of small bowel disease. A large volume of fluid is drunk to distend the small bowel. The fluid is high signal on T2-weighted images, so provides excellent visualization. Post-contrast T1-weighted scans show areas of abnormal bowel wall enhancement.

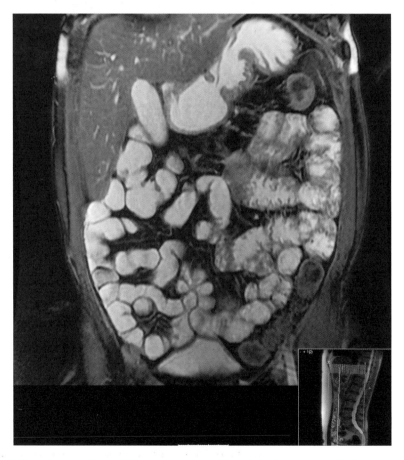

Normal T2-weighted small bowel MR images with good bowel distension, normal wall thickness and a normal fold pattern.

- Strictures can be identified as areas of bowel wall thickening that show abnormal contrast enhancement. There may be associated fistulae and abscesses.

The terminal ileal stricture is clearly depicted on MRI, which provides additional information on the bowel wall and extra-luminal anatomy. The traditional barium follow through provides information on the bowel lumen only.

- Ultrasound can demonstrate areas of bowel wall thickening, inflammatory change in the peri-intestinal fat, and fibro-fatty proliferation.

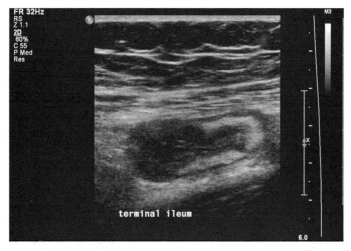

Ultrasound showing terminal ileitis, with low-density bowel wall thickening and loss of the normal wall layers indicating transmural inflammation.

- CT involves a radiation burden to the patient, which is undesirable in young patients, especially since repeated examinations are often necessary over a number of years.
- Other diseases affecting the terminal ileum include tuberculosis, *Yersinia* infection and lymphoma.

CLINICAL HOT LIST

- Incidence: 10–25 : 100,000 in the childhood population. Up to 40% of Crohn's disease presents before the age of 20.
- Presentation depends on the site of involvement (any part of the GI tract). The classical triad of colicky abdominal pain, diarrhoea and weight loss occurs in only 25%. Subtle presentations may occur with oropharyngeal or perianal disease. Other features include lethargy, poor growth, anorexia, fever, nausea, vomiting or extra-intestinal problems such as erythema nodosum, delayed puberty or arthropathy.
- Management aims to induce and maintain remission of disease, and to restore normal growth and nutrition. Strategies include steroids, 5-aminosalicylates, antibiotics, immunosuppression and exclusive enteral diets. Occasionally surgery is necessary but it is not curative.

FURTHER READING

Beattie RM, Croft NM, Fell JM et al. 2006: Inflammatory bowel disease. *Arch Dis Child;* 91: 426–32.

Darge A, Anupindi SA, Jaramillo D. 2008: MR imaging of the bowel: Pediatric applications. *Magn Reson Imaging Clin N Am;* 16: 467–78.

Toma P, Granata C, Magnano G, Barabino A. 2007: CT and MRI of paediatric Crohn disease. *Pediatr Radiol;* 37: 1083–92.

Case 75

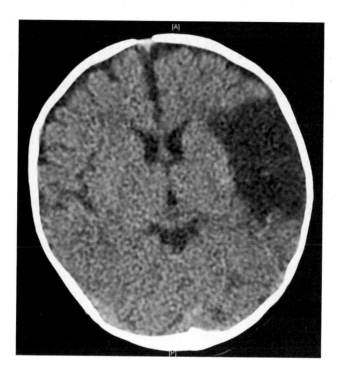

This 4-month-old baby has frequent seizures.

1. What does the CT brain show?
2. What is the diagnosis?

ANSWERS

1. There is a wedge-shaped area of low attenutation in the left frontal and temporal lobes indicating focal cerebral loss. There is no midline shift.
2. An established left middle cerebral artery territory infarct.

RADIOLOGY HOT LIST

- Brain infarction may result from occlusion of one (focal) or more (multifocal) vascular territories. The specific vascular distribution distinguishes vascular occlusive disease from the more generalized changes seen with hypoxic ischaemic encephalopathy (HIE) due to circulatory arrest.
- Occlusive brain infarction results in a wedge-shaped abnormality that is usually low density on CT involving the cortex in a specific vascular territory. HIE results in diffuse brain swelling, decreased grey/white matter differentiation and generalized low density of the cerebral white matter.
- Early cerebral infarction (< 24 hours) may not be visible on CT, or may be extremely subtle. MRI shows early ischaemic changes, with white matter oedema and restricted diffusion on diffusion-weighted images.
- Cranial ultrasound is useful in neonates, where ischaemic change may manifest as an area of non-specific increased echogenecity.
- Established infarction results in focal cerebral loss (gliosis) with consequent enlargement of the adjacent CSF spaces (prominent cerebral sulci and focal ventriculomegaly).
- Stroke in older children is usually due to arterial occlusion or haemorrhage.

CLINICAL HOT LIST

- Acute cerebral infarct is a rare but devastating diagnosis with far-reaching physical, emotional and social consequences. Frequently there is an underlying predisposition—10% of those with sickle cell anaemia will have a stroke.
- Causes of occlusive stroke in children include cardiac causes (congenital heart disease, myocarditis, valve disease), intracranial causes (vascular anomalies, arterial dissection, Moya Moya disease, sickle cell disease, vasculitis), and hypercoagulable states, particularly dehydration, meningoencephalitis, and radiation- and chemotherapy-induced stroke.
- HIE usually occurs secondary to circulatory collapse, of which there are cardiac and non-cardiac causes. Other causes include near drowning and strangulation.

FURTHER READING

Baumer JH. 2004: Childhood arterial stroke. *Arch Dis Child Ed Pract;* 89: ep50–3.
Bernard TJ, Goldenberg NA. 2008: Pediatric arterial ischemic stroke. *Pediatr Clin N Am;* 55: 323–338.

Case 76

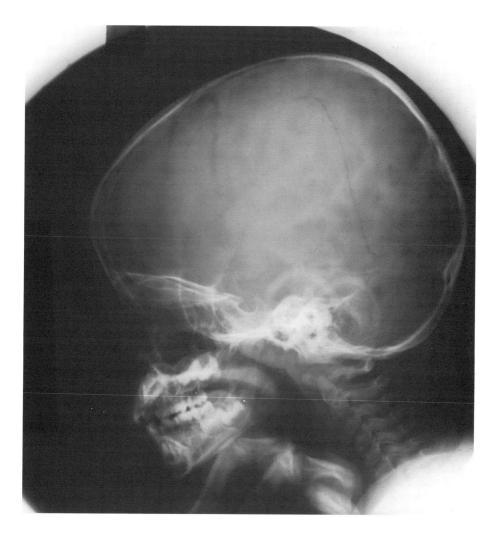

This 1-year-old boy was admitted after falling from his highchair at home.

1. What does the lateral skull X-ray show?

ANSWERS

1. There is a lucent line across the parietal bone, indicating a parietal skull fracture.

RADIOLOGY HOT LIST

- It is often difficult to differentiate between fractures, vascular markings and sutures.
- Fractures are usually straight lucent lines. Suture lines are interdigitated and in characteristic locations. Vascular markings usually have a tortuous and branching course.
- Depressed fractures usually appear as dense straight sclerotic lines.

FEATURES OF SKULL FRACTURES THAT ARE SUSPICIOUS OF NON-ACCIDENTAL HEAD INJURY

1. Complex fractures involving both sides of the skull.
2. Multiple fractures.
3. Widened fractures.
4. Depressed fractures, especially occipital.
5. Fractures that cross suture lines.
6. Growing fractures (traumatic encephaloceles).
7. No appropriate history from carer.

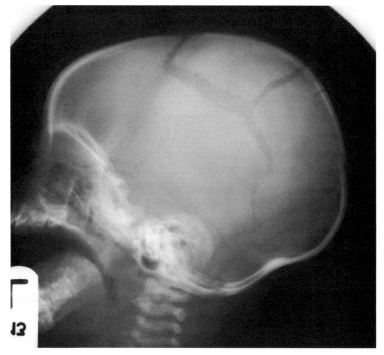

Skull fracture in NAI.

CLINICAL HOT LIST

- CT is the preferred imaging modality for head injury, as it is imperative to exclude intracranial injury. It involves a higher radiation dose than plain films and skull fractures can sometimes be more difficult to identify.
- Simple skull fractures in accidental trauma have a very low risk of intracranial sequelae. They usually involve falls from short distances, which impart a linear force to the head.
- A detailed history is mandatory, as a simple skull fracture remains the most common injury seen in non-accidental head trauma.

FURTHER READING

National Institute of Clinical Excellence. 2007: Clinical Guideline CG56. Head injury: triage, assessment, investigation and early management of head injury in infants, children and adults. http://www.nice.org.uk.

Case 77

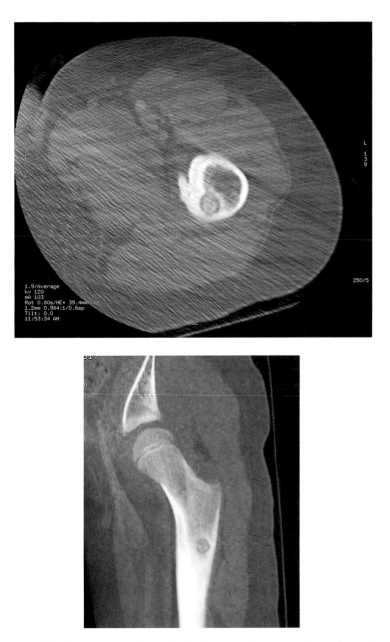

This 9-year-old girl has a painful left thigh. She is woken at night by the pain, which is only relieved by taking anti-inflammatory analgesia. A CT scan with axial and sagittal reconstructions has been acquired.

1. What does the CT scan of the right proximal femur show?
2. What is the most likely diagnosis?

ANSWERS

1. There is cortical thickening of the posterior cortex of the left proximal femur. This is associated with a well-defined lucent lesion that contains some central calcification.
2. Osteoid osteoma.

RADIOLOGY HOT LIST

- The classical description of an osteoid osteoma is a cortically based sclerotic lesion in a long bone, containing a small lucency (the nidus).
- The nidus causes pain and the surrounding reactive sclerosis.
- The nidus is lucent, but can develop some calcification within it. It then looks like a sequestrum as seen in osteomyelitis, which can be radiographically indistinguishable.
- Plain films may show an area of cortical thickening or sclerosis at the site of the lesion, with a small lucency. Bone scans show avid tracer uptake corresponding to the site of sclerosis.
- CT will demonstrate the exact location of the nidus, for both diagnosis and surgical planning or radiofrequency ablation.

CLINICAL HOT LIST

- A benign osteoblastic tumour, consisting of an osteoid-rich nidus in loose connective tissue, usually measuring 2 cm in diameter. They normally occur in those in the < 25 age group.
- They can occur anywhere, but > 80% are in the cortex of the shaft of long bones. The spine can be affected.
- The symptoms will vary with site but include localized deep pain (nocturnal or continuous), occasional swelling or tenderness and sometimes neurological symptoms.
- Treatment is with non-steroidal anti-inflammatory drugs (NSAIDs). Surgery is needed for intolerance to medication and failure to respond to therapy. Minimally invasive surgery is preferred to open resection.

FURTHER READING

Frassica FJ, Waltrip RL, Sponseller PD et al. 1996: Clinicopathologic features and treatment of osteoid osteoma and osteoblastoma in children and adolescents. *Orthop Clin North Am;* 27: 559–74.

Case 78

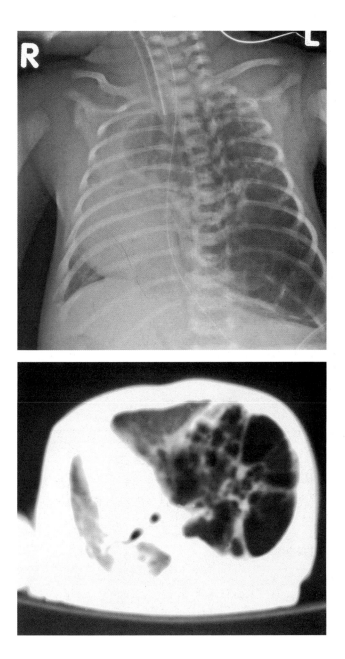

This baby was born at a specialist unit because of an antenatally diagnosed condition, and ventilated from birth.

1. What abnormalities are seen on the chest radiograph and CT scan?
2. What is the diagnosis?

ANSWERS

1. There are multiple large cystic spaces within the left hemithorax that are causing mass effect with mediastinal shift. They do not extend below the diaphragm. The tip of the nasogastric tube lies below the diaphragm.
2. Congenital cystic adenomatoid malformation.

RADIOLOGY HOT LIST

- It is typically an expansile cystic mass (almost always unilateral) with well-defined margins. It is usually fluid filled initially, and becomes lucent as air replaces the fluid.
- Mediastinal shift and compression of adjacent lung (with resultant pulmonary hypoplasia) are common. The bowel gas pattern is normal.
- It is often detected antenatally, but may regress during the course of pregnancy and be barely detectable at birth. In this case postnatal imaging should include ultrasound or CT scan as the CXR may appear normal.
- The differential diagnosis is a congenital diaphragmatic hernia.
- The three types of congenital cystic adenomatoid malformation are described as follows:

Type	Incidence	Appearance	Prognosis
Type 1	50%	Single/multiple large cysts > 20 mm)	Excellent with surgical resection
Type 2	40%	Multiple cysts (5–20 mm)	Poor—may be associated with congenital abnormalities
Type 3	10%	Large solid mass with no macroscopic cysts	Poor—due to associated pulmonary hypoplasia

CLINICAL HOT LIST

- This is a congenital hamartomatous lesion, which communicates with the bronchial tree and has a normal arterial supply and venous drainage. The characteristic cystic appearance develops postnatally as air-trapping occurs within the abnormal pulmonary tissue.
- The lesion is associated with a high mortality: 25% are stillborn; 20% have other congenital abnormalities (cardiac, renal, chromosomal anomalies).
- Potential antenatal interventions include aspiration, cystoamniotic shunt and fetal lobectomy.
- Surgical excision of lesions is recommended to prevent infection and because of the small risk of malignant transformation.

FURTHER READING

Paterson A. 2005: Imaging evaluation of congenital lung abnormalities in infants and children. *Radiol Clin N Am;* 43: 303–23.

Case 79

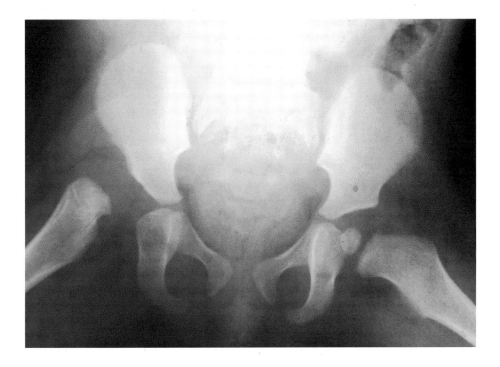

A 9-month-old baby has been noticed to have asymmetrical thigh creases and limb length discrepancy.

1. What does the plain X-ray of the pelvis show?
2. What is the diagnosis?
3. Name three risk factors.

ANSWERS

1. The right femur is displaced upwards and laterally. The right femoral capital epiphysis is not seen (due to delayed ossification) and the acetabulum on this side is poorly developed (with steep angulation of the acetabular roof).
2. Developmental dysplasia of the right hip (DDH), resulting in dislocation.
3. Family history of DDH, breech position in utero (particularly extended breech), other congenital spinal and lower limb abnormalities such as arthrogryphosis and spina bifida.

RADIOLOGY HOT LIST

- The plain radiograph is useful after the femoral capital epiphysis has ossified (usually after 4–6 months).
- Prior to this, ultrasound is the investigation of choice (no radiation and good visualization of the cartilaginous femoral head and acetabulum). Ultrasound will assess the hip both morphologically and dynamically. It demonstrates the degree of coverage of the head by the acetabulum, and the angle of the acetabular roof (the alpha angle).
- There is a spectrum of ultrasound findings from mild dysplasia to frank dislocation. Most mildly dysplastic hips resolve on follow up.

CLINICAL HOT LIST

- Incidence 1 : 100 at birth, 1 : 1000 at 1 year, F > M, bilateral in 10%.
- There is a spectrum from dislocatable to frank dislocation at rest. Routine screening is performed clinically with Ortolani and Barlow tests, and selectively with ultrasound.
- The clinical manifestations depend on age: asymmetrical thigh or gluteal creases, leg length discrepancy, a positive Galeazzi sign (relative shortness of the femur with the hips and knees flexed), delayed walking, Trendelenburg or waddling gait.
- Management depends on age at detection: persistent dysplasia with or without dislocation requires closed reduction usually with a Pavlik harness for 3–6 months. After 6 months of age, or in those who fail to respond to closed reduction methods, open reduction/femoral osteotomy and an abduction plaster may be required.

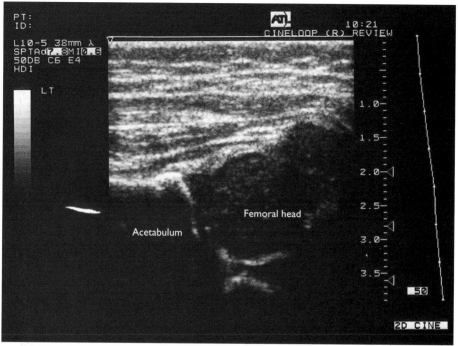

(a)

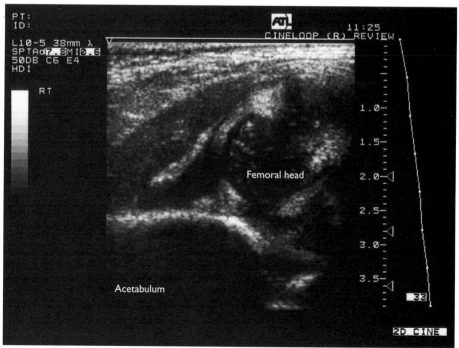

(b)

Ultrasound images of: (a) normal hip and (b) dislocated hip.

FURTHER READING

Committee on Quality Improvement, American Academy of Pediatrics. 2000: Clinical practice guidelines: Early detection of developmental dysplasia of the hip. *Pediatrics;* 105: 896–905.

Woolacott NF, Puhan MA, Steurer J, Kleijnen J. 2005: Ultrasonography in screening for developmental dysplasia of the hip in newborns: Systematic review. *BMJ;* 330: 1413–18.

Case 80

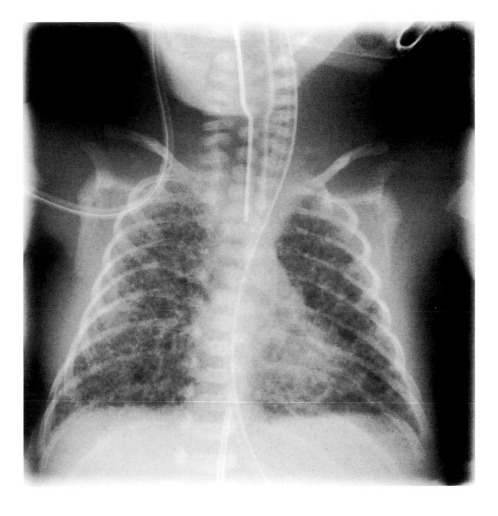

This 9-day-old neonate, born at 28 weeks' gestation, was ventilated for hyaline membrane disease (HMD).

1. What abnormality is seen on the chest radiograph?
2. What is the diagnosis?

ANSWERS

1. The lungs are hyperinflated (nine posterior ribs are visible and flattened diaphragms). Multiple, small, cystic air spaces are seen throughout both lungs. There is no pneumothorax. There is an endotracheal tube, a nasogastric tube and a umbilical artery catheter in situ.
2. Pulmonary interstitial emphysema (PIE).

RADIOLOGY HOT LIST

- PIE is a radiological diagnosis in an ill, ventilated neonate, usually with HMD, occasionally sepsis or meconium aspiration.
- The changes may be bilateral, but are often unilateral with mediastinal shift towards the unaffected side.
- Pneumothorax and pneumomediastinum are frequent complications.

CLINICAL HOT LIST

- PIE occurs predominantly as a consequence of mechanical ventilatation of neonates. Small airways rupture, causing air to leak into the bronchovascular sheaths.
- Changes of PIE occur within the first 2 weeks of life. Early presentation is associated with a worse prognosis, and is indicative of more severe underlying pulmonary disease.
- PIE is associated with high ventilator pressures, a misplaced endotracheal tube and other air leaks. It may lead to pulmonary hypertension and right-to-left ductal shunting. There is a high incidence of subsequent chronic lung disease.
- Management includes keeping pressures to a minimum and decompression stategies, e.g. nursing with the affected side down, pleurotomy, and selective intubation.

FURTHER READING

Agrons GA, Courtney SE, Stocker JT, Markowitz RI. 2005: From the Archives of the AFIP: Lung disease in premature neonates: Radiologic–pathologic correlation. *RadioGraphics;* 25: 1047–73.

Case 81

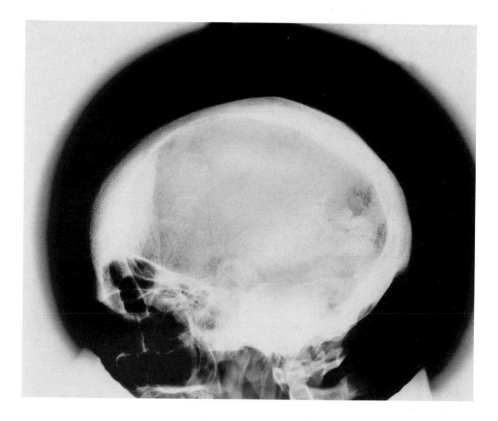

This 16-year-old male is under follow up for recurrent seizures. He has a 'birth mark' on the right side of his face, and a left hemiparesis.

1. List two abnormalities demonstrated on the lateral skull X-ray.
2. What is the diagnosis?

ANSWERS

1. There is serpiginous, tram-track calcification in the frontal and occipital region. The skull vault is markedly thickened.
2. Sturge–Weber syndrome.

RADIOLOGY HOT LIST

- Classical radiological appearances include gyriform intracranial calcification, cortical hemiatrophy with a thickened skull vault on the side of the angioma, and dilated ventricles with choroid plexus hypertrophy.
- Tram-track calcification following the contours of the gyri is not usually seen on plain radiographs until the age of 2 years. CT scans may show superficial cortical calcification at an earlier stage.

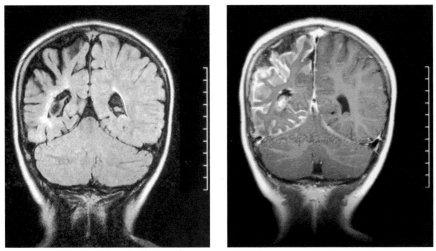

Pre- and post-enhancement T1-weighted MRI showing cortical atrophy of the right parietal and occipital lobes, and right meningeal enhancement. There is choroid plexus hypertrophy in the right lateral ventricle. There is some minor thickening of the right side of the vault.

CLINICAL HOT LIST

- A congenital vascular anomaly involving the eye, skin and brain.
- It is characterized by a port wine naevus of the face in the distribution of the trigeminal nerve (face and forehead), with a venous angioma of the ipsilateral cerebral meninges. These are thin-walled vessels within the pia mater.
- Clinical features include mental retardation, seizures (> 90%), contralateral hemiparesis and hemiatrophy and ipsilateral glaucoma.
- Management strategies include antiepileptic therapy and occasionally neurosurgical procedures for intractable epilepsy.

FURTHER READING

Comi AM. 2006: Advances in Sturge–Weber syndrome. *Curr Opin Neurol;* 19: 124–8.
Rastogi S, Lee C, Salamon N. 2008: Neuroimaging in pediatric epilepsy: A multimodality approach. *RadioGraphics;* 28: 1079–95.

Case 82

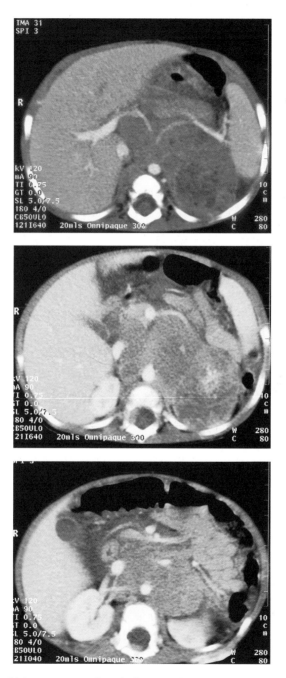

This 18-month-old boy presented with fever and weight loss. On examination, he was anaemic and had a palpable abdominal mass.

1. What abnormalities are shown on the contrast-enhanced CT scan of the abdomen?
2. What is the diagnosis?

ANSWERS

1. There is a large left suprarenal mass containing amorphous calcification and low-attenuation areas (consistent with central necrosis). It encases the aorta and coeliac axis, which is stretched anteriorly. The IVC is displaced to the right, whilst the left kidney is displaced inferiorly.
2. Neuroblastoma.

RADIOLOGY HOT LIST

- Neuroblastoma is the commonest extracranial malignant tumour of childhood.
- It arises in the abdomen in 60%, usually in the adrenal gland. 65% of patients have metastatic disease at presentation (bone, spinal canal, lymph nodes, lung and liver).
- Ultrasound will confirm the presence and location of an abdominal mass but CT/MRI is required for staging.
- Nuclear medicine scans (MIBG and bone scans) are performed to detect distant metastases, and to evaluate response to chemotherapy.
- Features distinguishing Wilms tumour from neuroblastoma:

Wilms	Neuroblastoma
Intrinsic renal mass	External compression/displacement of kidney
10% bilateral	Unilateral but usually crosses midline
< 10% contain calcification	85% contain calcification
Displaces vessels. Renal vein invasion in 5–10%	Vessel encasement

CLINICAL HOT LIST

- The tumour cells originate from the neural crest. The tumour can arise anywhere along the sympathetic chain or the adrenal medulla.
- Prognosis varies with age, staging and cytogenetic makeup.
- Treatment includes surgical resection, high-intensity chemotherapy, radiotherapy and autologous stem cell transplantation.
- Screening identifies more cases than would be expected, as some tumours resolve spontaneously.

FURTHER READING

Hildebrandt T, Traunecker H. 2005: Neuroblastoma: A tumour with many faces. *Curr Paed;* 15: 412–20.
Lonergan GJ, Schwab CM, Suarez ES, Carlson CL. 2002: From the Archives of the AFIP: Neuroblastoma, ganglioneuroblastoma, and ganglioneuroma: Radiologic–pathologic correlation. *RadioGraphics;* 22: 911–34.

Case 83

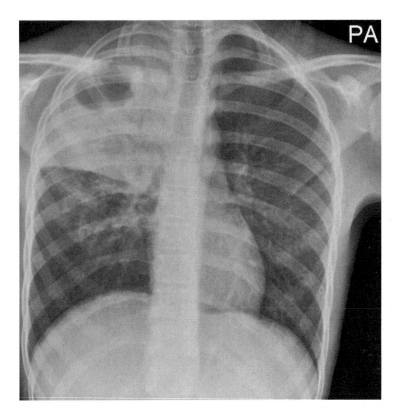

This 12-year-old boy is acutely unwell with fever and a productive cough. A CXR has been performed.

1. What does the CXR show?
2. What is the diagnosis?

ANSWERS

1. There is dense consolidation in the right upper lobe (the well-defined lower border represents the horizontal fissure), with air bronchograms visible adjacent to the right hilum. There is a large cavity within this.
2. Cavitating pnuemonia.

RADIOLOGY HOT LIST

- Consolidation (abnormal filling of the alveoli and air spaces) causes opacification of the lung, which may contain air bronchograms. In this case, the consolidation is limited by the horizontal fissure creating a well-defined inferior border, indicating that it is confined to the right upper lobe.
- The usual cause of lobar consolidation is pneumococcal infection, but the presence of cavitation suggests other micro-organisms such as *Staphlycoccus*, *Klebsiella*, gram-negative organisms and tuberculosis (TB).
- Lympadenopathy is the most common radiological finding in childhood primary TB. Reactivation TB is uncommon in children, and usually occurs in the upper lobes, often associated with cavitation.

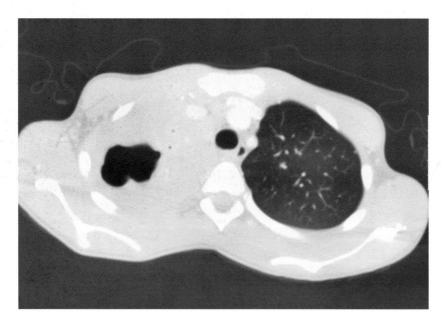

CT shows a large irregular cavity within the dense right upper lobe consolidation.

Case 84

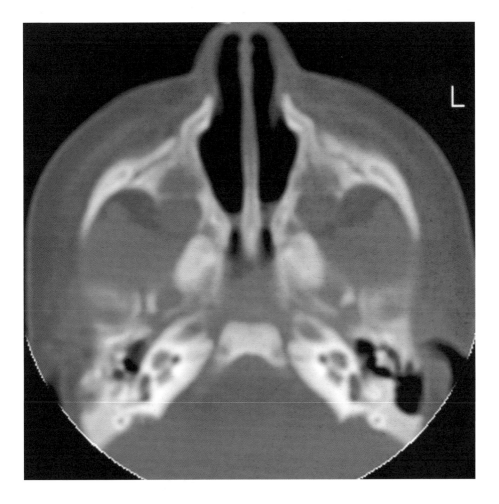

This 1-day-old term baby has tachypnoea and cyanosis during feeding. The midwives are unable to pass a nasogastric tube to facilitate top-up feeds.

1. What does the CT scan through the nasopharynx show?
2. What is the diagnosis?

ANSWERS

1. There are membranous septa occluding the posterior aspect of the nasal air passages bilaterally. The lateral walls of the nasal cavity are deviated medially.

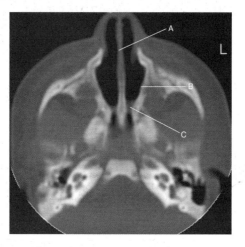

2. Bilateral membranous choanal atresia. A = nasal septum; B = lateral wall of nasal cavity; C = membraneous septum.

RADIOLOGY HOT LIST

- The occlusion may be bony (85%) or membranous (15%).
- A CT scan of the nasal airways (fine cuts) is the examination of choice—but the baby needs suction before the examination to ensure that retained secretions are not misinterpreted as membranous septa.

CLINICAL HOT LIST

- Incidence is 1 : 8000 and unilateral is more common than bilateral. 50% are associated with CHARGE syndrome (**C**oloboma, **H**eart disease, choanal **A**tresia, **R**etarded growth, **G**enital hypoplasia, **E**ar abnormalities). There is also an association with Treacher-Collins syndrome.
- It usually presents with apnoea, cyanosis, respiratory distress and feeding difficulties in a neonate. Unilateral atresia may present later with milder symptoms or nasal discharge.
- Babies are obligatory nose-breathers until 3 months of age, unless they are crying. These babies may therefore be pink when crying and distressed/dusky at rest.
- The diagnosis may be suspected by the inability to pass a nasogastric tube.
- The airway may require protection (oral airway or intubation) prior to definitive surgery.

FURTHER READING

Valencia MP, Castillo M. 2008: Congenital and acquired lesions of the nasal septum: A practical guide for differenial diagnosis. *RadioGraphics;* 28: 205–23.

Case 85

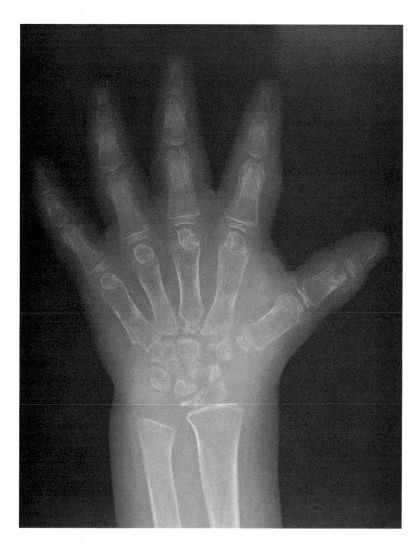

This 4-year-old boy has a painful left wrist.

1. What does the X-ray show?
2. What is the diagnosis?

ANSWERS

1. There is soft tissue swelling around the wrist. The bones are osteopenic. The carpal bones are small and irregular, with multiple erosions. There are further erosions of the bases of the second, third and fourth metacarpals and of many of the small joints. There is loss of the joint space at the radiocarpal and intercarpal joints.
2. Juvenile idiopathic arthritis (JIA).

RADIOLOGY HOT LIST

- The earliest signs in the wrist include periarticular osteopenia and soft tissue swelling. Later changes include erosions, periosteal reactions, joint space loss and joint destruction.
- Spinal changes include diffuse ankylosis of the posterior articular joints (especially in the cervical spine) and atlanto-axial subluxation.
- Hyperaemia of the affected joints may cause overgrowth of the epiphyses with premature closure of the growth plates (and therefore bone shortening).
- Gadolinium-enhanced MRI scans can detect synovial hypertrophy and acute synovitis.

CLINICAL HOT LIST

- JIA is defined as chronic arthritis (> 6 weeks) of unknown aetiology before the 16th birthday.
- Incidence is 1 : 10,000, prevalence 1 : 1000.
- Management is multidisciplinary. Medical treatment includes NSAIDs, steroids, methotrexate (IV, intra-articular or oral) and biologics, e.g. etanercept. Physiotherapy, occupational therapy, and psychological support are also employed. Early treatment helps prevent localized growth abnormalities, e.g. leg length discrepancy.
- Uveitis screening by an ophthalmologist is mandatory for all with JIA as chronic anterior uveitis is silent and sight threatening.

Systemic onset	Quotidian fever, evanescent erythematous rash, hepatosplenomegaly, lymphadenopathy and serositis may all preceed arthritis
Oligoarticular-persistent	4 or fewer joints affected often ANA + Associated with chronic anterior uveitis
Oligoarticular-extended	As above but > 4 joints involved after the first 6 months
Polyarticular RF positive	5 or more joints involved, similar to rheumatoid arthritis
Polyarticular RF negative	5 or more joints involved
Enthesitis-related arthritis (ERA)	Arthritis +/− enthesitis (inflammation at insertion of tendon/fascia/ligament into bone) HLA B27+, acute anterior uveitis, spinal inflammation
Psoriatic	With psoriasis/nail changes or dactylitis

FURTHER READING

Buchmann RF, Jaramillo D. 2004: Imaging of articular disorders in children. *Radiol Clin N Am;* 42: 151–68.

Case 86

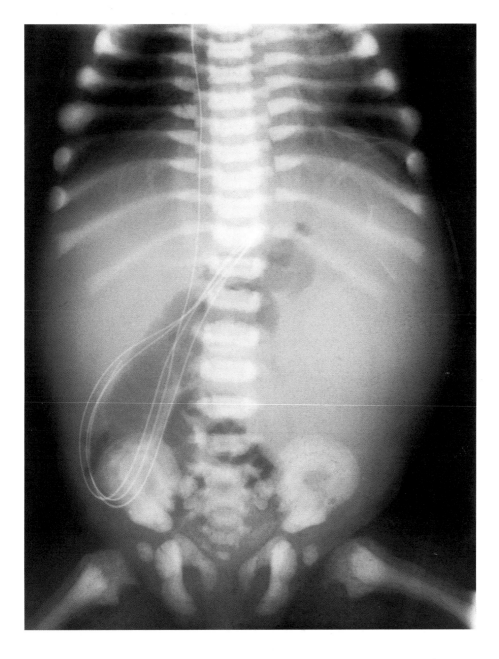

This 6-month-old baby has a rare inherited disorder. On examination he is found to have hepatosplenomegaly.

1. What abnormalities are seen on the X-ray?
2. What is the diagnosis?

244

ANSWERS

1. The bones are diffusely sclerotic, with obliteration of the normal trabecular pattern. There is a 'bone-within-a-bone' appearance best appreciated in the pelvis and proximal femora. There is displacement of the bowel gas by an enlarged liver and spleen.
2. Osteopetrosis (Albers-Schönberg disease).

RADIOLOGY HOT LIST

- A characteristic finding is diffuse osteosclerosis with cortical thickening and medullary encroachment. The bones appear dense with loss of the normal trabecular pattern. The 'bone-within-bone' appearance is classical.
- Though appearing sclerotic, the bones are actually brittle and weak—look for pathological fractures, which usually heal with exuberant callus formation.
- Osteosclerosis causes obliteration of the paranasal sinuses, mastoid air cells and skull base foramina.

CLINICAL HOT LIST

- This is a rare hereditary disorder with both recessive and dominant inheritance, the latter being clinically less severe.
- There is a failure of osteoclast resorption causing persistence of the cartilaginous and calcified bone matrix. The bones are abnormally sclerotic but structurally weak.
- Obliteration of the medullary cavity causes marrow depression with subsequent anaemia, leucocytopaenia, and thrombocytopaenia. Extramedullary haemopoiesis leads to hepatosplenomegaly.
- Bony overgrowth causes narrowing of the neural foramina, resulting in cranial nerve palsies. Optic atrophy and deafness are common findings in the recessive form. Presentation is commonly with visual problems, e.g. squint/roving eyes.
- In the recessive form survival beyond childhood is uncommon and death is usually due to haemorrhage, recurrent infection or leukaemia.
- Bone marrow transplantation (BMT) is potentially curative.

FURTHER READING

Wilson CJ, Vellodi A. 2000: Personal practice: Autosomal recessive osteopetrosis: diagnosis, management, and outcome. *Arch Dis Childhood;* 83: 449–52.

Case 87

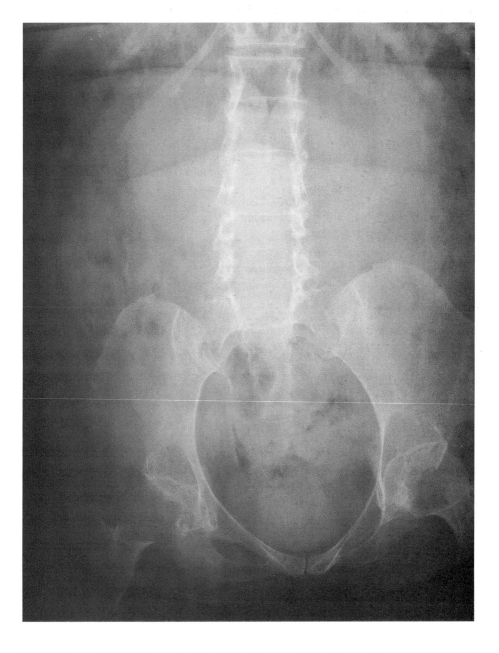

This 18-year-old girl is paraplegic, with urinary and faecal incontinence.

1. What does the X-ray of the lumbar spine show?
2. What is the diagnosis?

ANSWERS

1. The posterior elements of the lumbar spine are absent (absent laminae and spinous processes) with a widened spinal canal. Note the widening of the interpedicular distance.
2. Spina bifida.

RADIOLOGY HOT LIST

- Remember to assess the spine on a plain film of the abdomen! Identify the pedicles, laminae and spinous processes—if these are absent, or incompletely fused, a diagnosis of spinal dysraphism can be made.
- The diagnosis is often made by antenatal ultrasound (complex mass seen outside spinal canal with separation of the posterior laminae).
- There is a high incidence of associated hydrocephalus (usually detected antenatally).
- There may be other central nervous system (CNS) abnormalities including Arnold–Chiari malformation, intraspinal dermoid and lipoma, tethered cord and diastematomyelia. These can be further assessed with MRI. Ultrasound can be used to assess the spine in young babies.

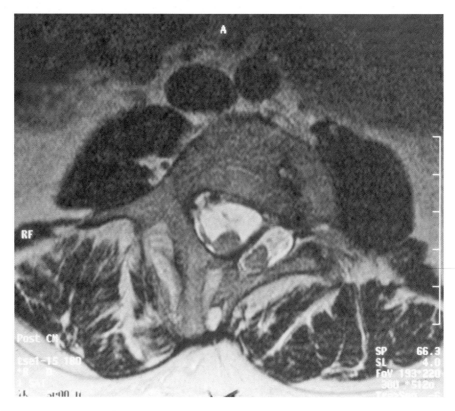

Diastomatomyelia. Axial T2-weighted MRI showing a fibrous septum dividing the bony spinal canal and spinal cord at L2, resulting in two hemicords.

CLINICAL HOT LIST

- Spinal dysraphism is a spectrum of disorders ranging from mildly deficient lumbar spinous processes (spina bifida occulta) to an open defect with exposed abnormal spinal cord and CSF leakage (spina bifida cystica).
- Clinical manifestations depend on the site and extent of the lesion. There may be complete loss of motor, sensory and reflex function below the affected level. Involvement of the sacral roots leads to bowel and bladder dysfunction.
- Neurosurgical repair aims to achieve a watertight closure of the defect without worsening the neurological status. Ventricular shunting may be required for hydrocephalus.
- Multidisciplinary management should include neurosurgical, orthopaedic and urological input as well as physiotherapy and occupational therapy assessment.
- Folic acid supplementation can reduce the incidence of neural tube defects by as much as 80%.

FURTHER READING

Kaufman BA. 2004: Neural tube defects. *Pediatr Clin North Am;* 51: 389–419.

Unsinn KM, Geley T, Freund MC, Gassner I. 2000: US of the spinal cord in newborns: Spectrum of normal findings, variants, congenital anomalies, and acquired diseases. *RadioGraphics;* 20: 923–38.

Case 88

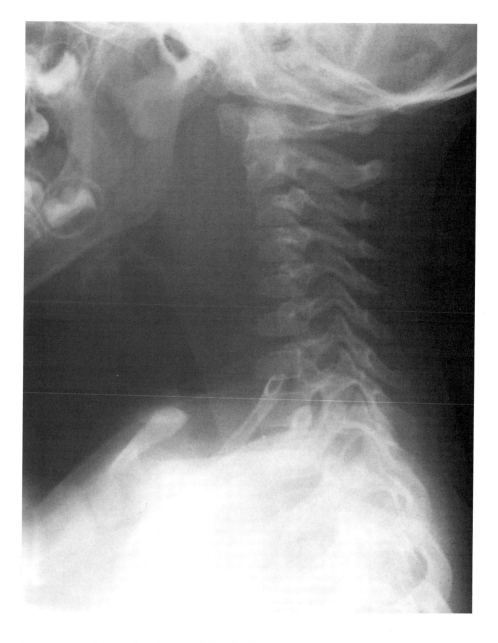

This 2-year-old boy has fever and dysphagia.

1. What abnormality is seen on the lateral X-ray of the neck?
2. What is the diagnosis?

ANSWERS

1. There is swelling of the prevertebral soft tissues with anterior displacement of the trachea. There is loss of the normal cervical lordosis but the bones appear normal.
2. Retropharyngeal abscess.

RADIOLOGY HOT LIST

- Swelling of the prevertebral soft tissues implies infection or haemorrhage. In a child the thickness of the normal prevertebral soft tissues is 3–5 mm between C1 and C4 (2–3 mm in an adult) and the width of the vertebral body below C4.
- There may be reversal of the normal cervical lordosis as the head is held in an abnormal position. Erosion of bone or disc height reduction indicates an underlying osteomyelitis or discitis.
- Gas or an air–fluid level in the retropharyngeal tissues is highly suggestive of an abscess.
- A CT scan will confirm the diagnosis in equivocal cases and define the superior and inferior mediastinal extent. This is particularly important if surgical drainage is contemplated.

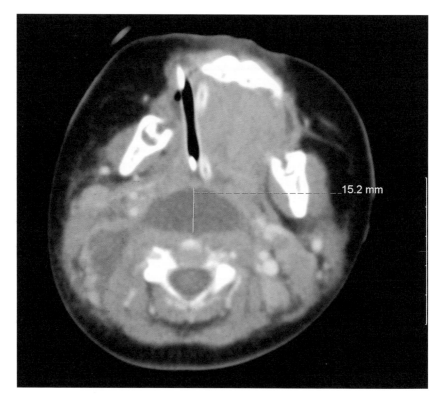

CT showing a retropharyngeal abscess in a ventilated child.

- The differential diagnosis includes haematoma, lymphadenopathy, and (rarely) neoplasm (rhabdomyosarcoma).

CLINICAL HOT LIST

- Rare infection of the posterior pharyngeal wall occurring in babies and young children between 6 months to 6 years.
- Aetiology: upper respiratory tract infection, extension of suppurative cervical lymphadenitis, or perforating injury of the pharynx or oesophagus.
- The child presents with fever, drooling and their head held back due to airway obstruction. Important differential diagnoses include epiglottitis and tonsillitis.
- Typical organisms: *Staphylococcus*, *Streptococcus*, mixed flora.
- The first priority of management is to protect a compromised airway. Intravenous antibiotics are usually required and surgical drainage may be needed.

Case 89

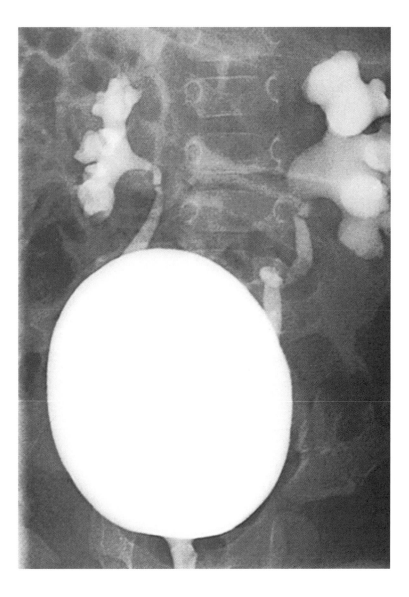

This 4-month-old girl had been treated for a urinary tract infection. A micturating cystourethrogram was performed as part of her investigations.

1. What abnormalities are seen?
2. What is the diagnosis?

ANSWERS

1. Contrast has refluxed into dilated collecting systems and ureters bilaterally. The renal calyces are clubbed.
2. Bilateral vesicoureteric reflux (VUR).

RADIOLOGY HOT LIST

- There is still controversy over the strategy for investigation of urinary tract infection, with debate over the choice of investigation used to detect reflux and the age group that should be investigated. There is thus local variation in practice.
- A contrast MCUG is recommended in boys where visualization of the urethra is important in order to exclude posterior urethral valves.
- When possible, girls can have a direct nuclear medicine cystogram, as images of the urethra are not required. Beyond the age of 3, most children can micturate on request. Nuclear medicine studies then become the investigation of choice, with a reduction in radiation dose, and a more pleasant experience for all concerned.
- Grading of reflux:

Grade	Characteristics
1	Reflux to ureter, but not kidney
2	Reflux into non-dilated ureter, pelvis, and calyces
3	Reflux to calyces with mild dilatation
4	Reflux to calyces, with moderate dilatation and clubbed calyces
5	Gross dilatation and tortuous ureters

CLINICAL HOT LIST

- MCUG is recommended after atypical or recurrent UTI in those aged < 6/12 years, or if there is an abnormal USS or a positive family history in those < 3 years of age.
- There is an important association between UTI, VUR, renal scarring, hypertension and chronic renal failure. Most cases of VUR resolve spontaneously.
- Management (prophylactic antibiotics, frequent voiding, treatment of constipation) aims to prevent renal scarring by prevention of UTI. Parental vigilance for UTI symptoms and regular assessment of renal growth and possible scarring are essential.
- Surgical management, including ureteric reimplantation, is reserved for failure of medical management, complex abnormalities and obstruction.

FURTHER READING

Coulthard MG. 2008: Is reflux nephropathy preventable, and will the NICE childhood UTI guidelines help? *Arch Dis Childhood;* 93: 196–9.

Riccabona M, Avni FE, Blickman JG. 2008: Imaging recommendations in paediatric uroradiology: minutes of the ESPR workgroup session on urinary tract infection, fetal hydronephrosis, urinary tract ultrasonography and voiding cystourethrography. *Pediatr Radiol;* 38: 138–45.

Case 90

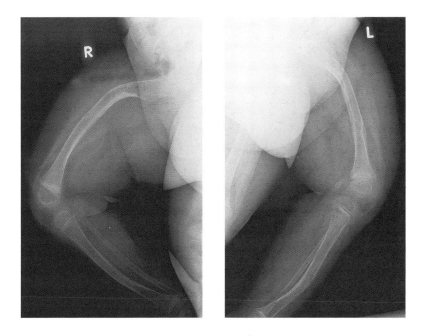

This 18-month-old girl has had multiple admissions after minor trauma.

1. What do the X-rays of the legs show?
2. What is the diagnosis?

ANSWERS

1. The bones are osteopenic with cortical thinning and modelling deformities (markedly bowed). There is a breach in the cortex of the left femoral shaft associated with a periosteal reaction, indicating a recent fracture.
2. Osteogenesis imperfecta.

RADIOLOGY HOT LIST

- Radiographic features of osteogenesis imperfecta include generalized cortical thinning, with gracile bones. The proximal humeri and femora may be expanded. There are usually bowing deformities present.
- Fractures are common, and they may heal with exuberant callus formation. Operative interventions (osteotomy and internal pinning) are frequent.
- There may be Wormian (intrasutural) bones in the skull, and a thin calvarium. Kyphoscoliosis and vertebral scalloping are a common finding in the spine. The pelvis may show protrusio acetabulae.

CLINICAL HOT LIST

- These are a group of inherited disorders of defective production of type I collagen.
- The management includes prevention of fractures, IV bisphosphonates (reduce fracture frequency and pain) orthopaedic surgery, nutrition (calcium/vitamin D) and physiotherapy.

Type	Inheritance	Clinical manifestations
I	AD	Commonest form, with pathological fractures as a toddler, blue sclerae, hypotonia, hypermobility, deafness, abnormal teeth
II	New dominant mutation	Multiple intrauterine fractures with death in utero
III	AD/AR	Multiple fractures from infancy, severe progressive skeletal deformities, kyphoscoliosis, chest deformities, premature death from respiratory failure
IV	AD	Bone disease similar to type I, but manifestations are less severe than types II and III

FURTHER READING

Åström E. 2008: Management of osteogenesis imperfecta. *Paediatr Child Health;* 18: 97–8.

Case 91

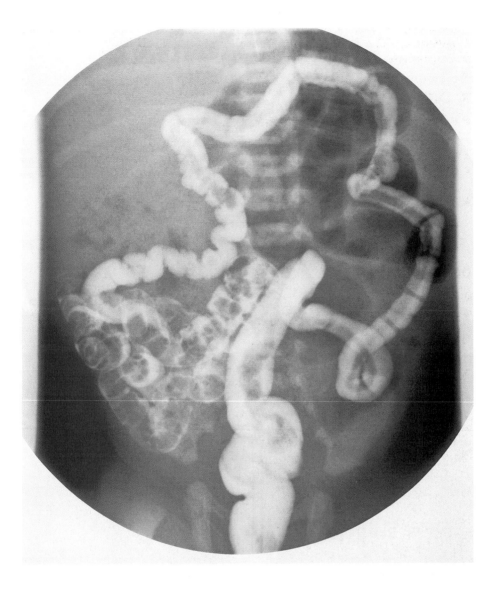

This 3-day-old baby was brought to A & E with vomiting, abdominal distension and failure to pass meconium. The plain abdominal radiograph showed multiple dilated loops of bowel. A contrast enema was performed.

1. List three abnormalities demonstrated on the enema.
2. What is the likely diagnosis?
3. What is the associated condition?

ANSWERS

1. There is a narrow calibre empty colon (microcolon). There are dilated loops of small bowel, and the distal ileum contains large filling defects, which are meconium plugs.
2. Meconium ileus.
3. Cystic fibrosis.

RADIOLOGY HOT LIST

- A contrast enema is the investigation of choice in low bowel obstruction.
- In this case, contrast refluxes back into the terminal ileum, which appears larger than the colon. The ileum contains multiple rounded filling defects due to masses of inspissated meconium.
- Distinguish this appearance from meconium plug syndrome, which is a functional motility disorder of the bowel and not associated with cystic fibrosis. A contrast enema in this condition shows a large filling defect in the rectum and colon due to a long meconium cast.
- Both conditions may be treated with a therapeutic enema to relieve the obstruction (this is successful in 50% of cases of meconium ileus; the other 50% will require surgery).

CLINICAL HOT LIST

- Meconium ileus is almost always associated with cystic fibrosis. The meconium is thick and viscid, occluding small bowel and not passing distally. The associated microcolon is of normal length and orientation but narrow calibre. It is unused, containing no (or very little) meconium.
- 10% of cystic fibrosis patients present with neonatal intestinal obstruction.
- Distal intestinal obstruction syndrome (DIOS), sometimes referred to as 'meconium ileus equivalent', has a similar pathophysiology to meconium ileus and occurs in older children and adults with cystic fibrosis.
- Meconium plug syndrome is a neonatal functional motility disorder.

FURTHER READING

Smyth RL. 2005: Diagnosis and management of cystic fibrosis. *Arch Dis Child Ed Pract;* 90: ep1–6.

Newman B. 1999: Imaging of neonatal gastrointestinal obstruction. *Radiol Clin N Am;* 37: 1049–65.

Case 92

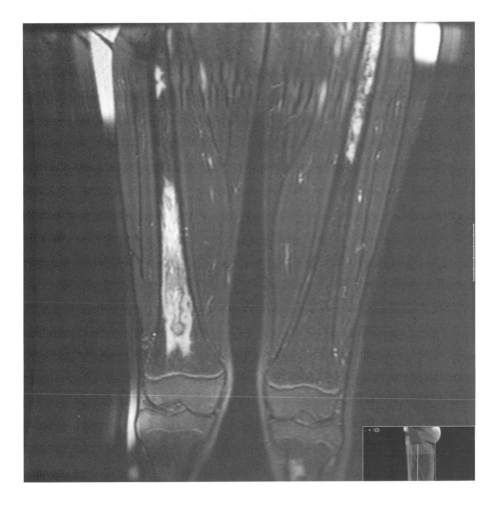

This 8-year-old Afro-Caribbean girl was admitted to the ward with acute severe bilateral leg pain. She has an underlying haematological condition. An MRI scan of her lower limbs was performed.

1. What abnormality is seen on the T2-weighted, fat-saturated MRI scan?
2. What is the most likely diagnosis?

ANSWERS

1. There are large focal areas of high signal within the bone marrow of both femoral shafts. These show serpiginous low-signal margins. There is no associated periosteal reaction or soft tissue oedema.
2. Acute bone infarcts complicating sickle cell disease.

RADIOLOGY HOT LIST

- Acute bone infarcts cause marked bone marrow oedema. In a fat-saturated T2 MRI image, the marrow fat should appear dark. The area of oedema stands out as a bright high-signal area, with surrounding low-density serpiginous lines. The area will appear as low signal on T1-weighted images.
- The differential is osteomyelitis, where there may be a periosteal reaction, subperiosteal collections and adjacent soft tissue oedema.
- The anatomical distribution of blood vessels supplying the vertebra results in focal infarction affecting the central part of the vertebral body. This causes central depression of the end-plates, giving the characteristic 'H-shaped' vertebral body.

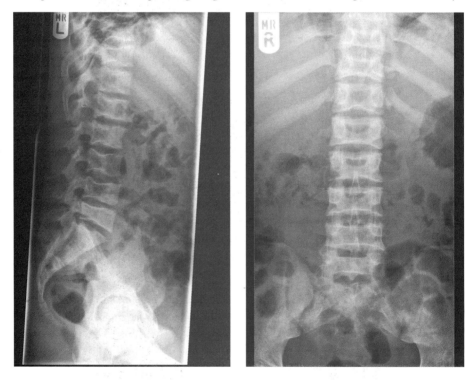

AP and lateral lumbar spine X-rays show typical 'H- shaped' vertebral bodies.

- Cardiomegaly may occur due to haemosiderotic cardiomyopathy (repeated transfusions causing iron overload) or high-output cardiac failure.
- Sickle chest syndrome comprises changes of pulmonary infarction and subsequent consolidation. Rapid widespread change is suggestive of sickle chest syndrome. The differential diagnosis for consolidation in sickle cell disease is pneumococcal pneumonia, which classically causes lobar consolidation.

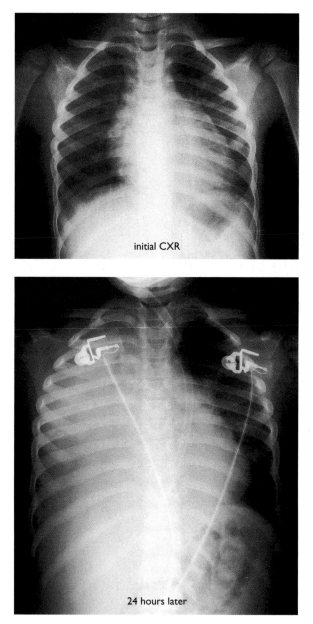

The initial chest radiograph shows cardiomegaly but there is rapid progression to right lung consolidation over 24 hours, which is suggestive of acute sickle chest syndrome.

CLINICAL HOT LIST

- Sickle cell disease is a chronic haemolytic anaemia with intermittent symptoms due to infarction, sequestration and infection. These may be precipitated by the cold, infection, dehydration and acidosis.
- Clinical presentations are as follows:

Dactylitis	Infantile presentation affecting hands and feet
Splenic sequestration	Rapid life-threatening hypovolaemic shock caused by extensive red cell trapping in spleen
Painful crisis	Widespread microvascular occlusion usually in long bones or back
Aplastic crisis	Reticulocyte failure due to parvovirus or folate deficiency
Neurological crisis	Acute stroke, intracerebral sickling
Infection	Bacteraemia or osteomyelitis secondary to *Pneumococcus*, *Haemophilus*, or *Salmonella*
Chest syndrome	Pulmonary infarction

- Management strategies: parental education, penicillin prophylaxis, hydroxyurea, transfusion programmes and avoidance of crisis precipitants.
- Management of an acute crisis includes oxygen, hydration, analgesia and antibiotics. Exchange transfusion may be required for chest and neurological crises. Immediate transfusion is indicated for splenic sequestration.

FURTHER READING

Howard J, Davies SC. 2007: Haemoglobinopathies. *Paediatr Child Health;* 17: 311–16.
Madani G, Papadopoulou AM, Holloway B et al. 2007: The radiological manifestations of sickle cell disease. *Clin Radiol;* 62: 528–38.

Case 93

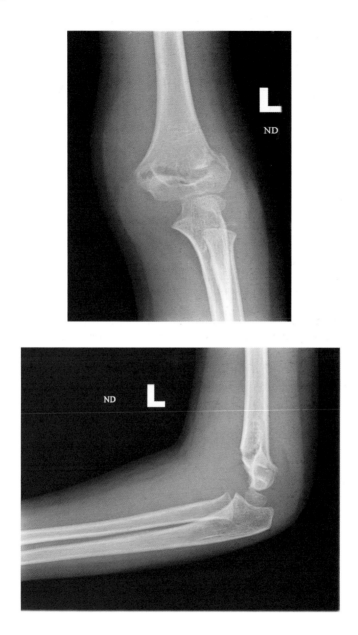

This 5-year-old boy came into the A & E department after falling off his scooter.

1. What does the X-ray show?

ANSWERS

1. The anterior and posterior fat pads are elevated, indicating a joint effusion. There is a supracondylar fracture, with a transverse lucency clearly seen on the AP film.

RADIOLOGY HOT LIST

- Supracondylar fractures are easily overlooked. Always check the fat pads on the lateral view of the elbow. There is a joint effusion present if they are elevated, which is highly suggestive of an intra-articular fracture. If the fracture is not visible, follow-up films are indicated.
- Any disruption of the cortex is suspicious. If the fracture is displaced it will normally disrupt the anterior humeral line (see diagram), which should pass through the middle third of the capitellum.

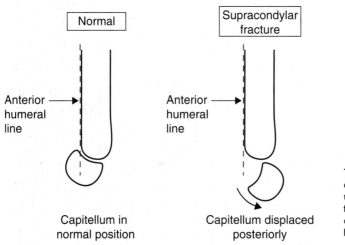

Normal	Supracondylar fracture
Anterior humeral line	Anterior humeral line
Capitellum in normal position	Capitellum displaced posteriorly

The capitellum is displaced posteriorly due the supracondylar fracture, causing disruption of the anterior humeral line.

CLINICAL HOT LIST

- This is the commonest elbow fracture in childhood. The average age is 6–7 years, and it is rare after 15 years.
- It is usually caused by a fall on the outstretched hand.
- It can be complicated by neurovascular injury:
  —up to 10% will temporarily lose the radial pulse due to swelling.
  —median, radial or anterior interosseous nerves may be involved.
- Management will depend on displacement and vascular compromise—it varies from splinting to manipulation under anaesthetic and pinning.
- The outcome is usually very good, with complete resolution of motor and sensory deficit on conservative management only.

FURTHER READING

Morewood DJ. 1987: Incidence of unsuspected fractures in traumatic effusions of the elbow joint. *Br Med J (Clin Res Ed);* 295: 109–10.

CASE 94

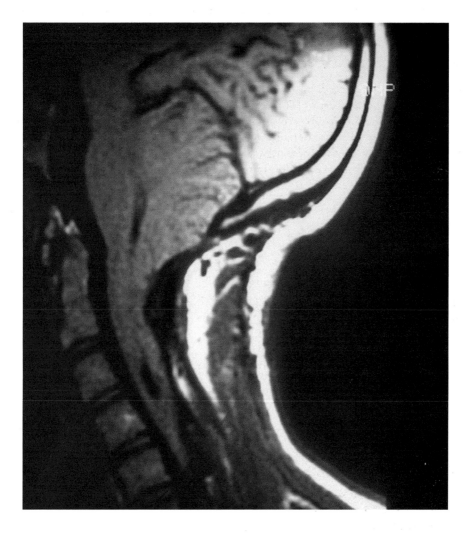

This 14-year-old girl has a lumbar myelomeningocele.

1. What abnormalities are seen on the (T1-weighted) midline sagittal MRI scan?
2. What is the diagnosis?

ANSWERS

1. The cerebellar tonsils and vermis are herniated through the foramen magnum, with an elongated and caudally displaced IVth ventricle. There is a syrinx in the cervical cord.
2. Arnold–Chiari type II malformation.

RADIOLOGY HOT LIST

- The characteristic radiological findings in Arnold–Chiari type II malformation are hindbrain dygenesis with a caudally displaced IVth ventricle and brainstem, and herniation of the cerebellar tonsils through the foramen magnum.
- The degree of abnormality can vary widely from patient to patient.
- Associations include:

Spinal anomalies	Lumbar myelomeningoceles (> 95%), syringomyelia
Supratentorial anomalies	Obstructive hydrocephalus, dysgenesis of the corpus callosum, excessive cortical gyration

- Arnold–Chiari type I (mild herniation of the cerebellar tonsils) is a frequent isolated finding, often of little clinical significance and without associated supratentorial abnormalities.

CLINICAL HOT LIST

- Clinical manifestations include hydrocephalus, lower limb spasticity, upper limb weakness, Erb's palsy, neck pain, lower cranial nerve palsies (due to downward displacement of the medulla) and respiratory abnormalities (brainstem compression).
- Neurosurgical management may be required to decompress the foramen magnum.

Case 95

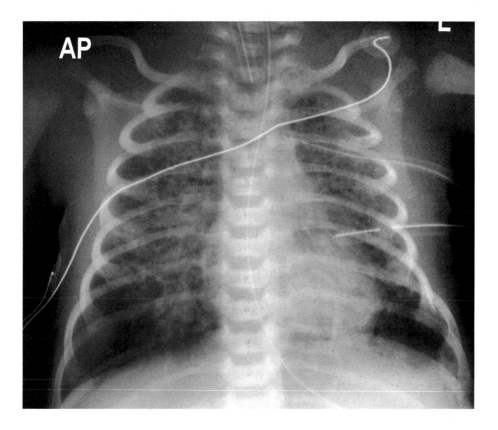

This term baby is being ventilated on the neonatal unit after an emergency Caesarean section for fetal distress.

1. What abnormalities are seen on the chest radiograph?
2. What is the most likely diagnosis?

ANSWERS

1. The lungs are hyperinflated with flattened hemidiaphragms. There are bilateral, coarse, patchy infiltrates in both lungs, with areas of air trapping at both bases. Two intercostal drains are present in the left hemithorax, but there is no residual pneumothorax.
2. Meconium aspiration syndrome (MAS).

RADIOLOGY HOT LIST

- Meconium aspiration causes obstruction of the airways, resulting in hyperinflation and areas of atelectasis and air trapping. Radiographic appearances depend on the severity of the aspiration.
- Look for pneumothorax and pneumomediastinum (seen in 25% of cases).
- Radiographic appearances may be indistinguishable from neonatal pneumonia and pulmonary haemorrhage.

CLINICAL HOT LIST

- This disorder occurs because of fetal asphyxia in term and postmature neonates:

Meconium	Pulmonary effects
Highly viscous	Ball-valve effect causes air trapping
Chemical irritant	Pneumonitis
Opposes surfactant	Reduces lung compliance
Associated with chorioamnionitis	Pneumonia

- Treatment of established MAS is based on respiratory support with conventional mechanical ventilation and surfactant therapy.
- A major complication is persistent pulmonary hypertension. This may necessitate high-frequency oscillation ventilation, nitric oxide or extracorporeal membrane oxidation (ECMO).

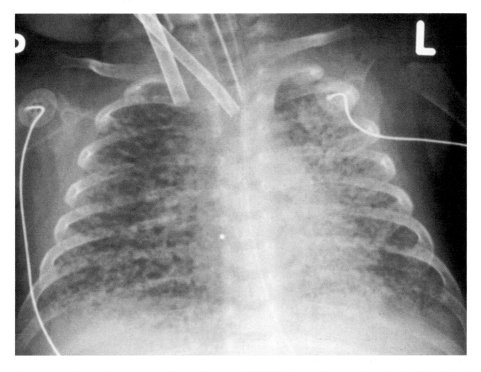

Severe meconium aspiration treated by ventilation and ECMO (via two large catheters in the right side of the neck).

- It is associated with hypoxic ischaemic encephalopathy and renal failure.

FURTHER READING

Ibrahim CPH, Subheda NV. 2005: Management of meconium aspiration syndrome. *Curr Paed;* 15: 92–8.

Newman B. 1999: Imaging of medical disease of the newborn lung. *Radiol Clin N Am;* 37: 1049–65.

Case 96

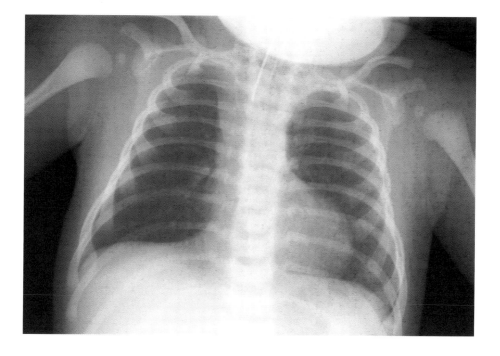

This 1-day-old baby is cyanotic.

1. What does the CXR show?
2. What is the diagnosis?

ANSWERS

1. There is a boot-shaped heart. The cardiac apex is elevated (right ventricular hypertrophy) and the pulmonary bay is concave due to a hypoplastic main pulmonary artery. The lungs are relatively oligaemic. The endotracheal tube is in a satisfactory position.
2. Tetralogy of Fallot.

RADIOLOGY HOT LIST

- Tetralogy of Fallot has a typical radiographic appearance due to right ventricular hypertrophy and underdevelopment of the main pulmonary artery. There may be a right-sided aortic arch in 25%.
- Evaluate the pulmonary vascularity on the CXR: this will narrow the differential diagnosis in the assessment of cyanotic congenital heart disease.
- CXR appearances in cyanotic congenital heart disease are:

Pulmonary vascularity	Causes
Increased	Transposition of the great arteries, truncus arteriosus, total anomalous pulmonary venous drainage, single ventricle
Decreased with normal heart size	Tetralogy of Fallot
Decreased with cardiomegaly	Ebstein's anomaly, pulmonary atresia, tricuspid atresia

CLINICAL HOT LIST

- Fallot's tetralogy is the commonest congenital cyanotic cardiac lesion (6% of all congenital heart malformations).
- The tetralogy comprises a ventricular septal defect, pulmonary stenosis, overriding aorta and right ventricular hypertrophy.
- It presents with cyanosis (severe defects present early). Hypercyanotic spells may occur due to infundibular spasm.
- Surgery is the definitive treatment: either a one-stage repair or an initial palliative procedure (Blalock–Taussig shunt) followed by repair.
- Medical complications include high haematocrit, hyperviscosity and infective endocarditis.

FURTHER READING

Barnes N, Archer N. 2005: Understanding congenital heart disease. *Curr Paed;* 15: 421–8.

Strife JL, Sze RW. 1999: Radiographic evaluation of neonate with congenital heart disease. *Radiol Clin N Am;* 37: 1093–107.

Case 97

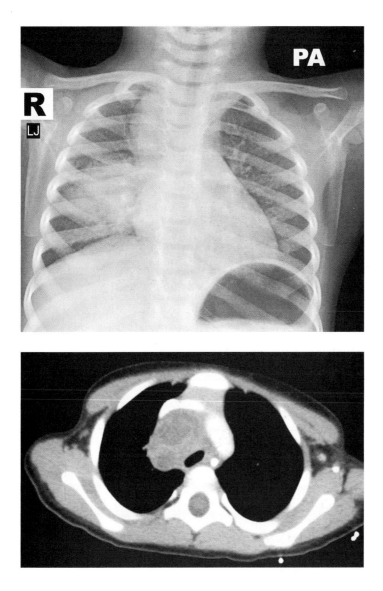

This 3-year-old Bangladeshi boy was seen by his GP for persistent cough, fever and failure to thrive.

1. What do his CXR and CT scan show?
2. What is the most likely diagnosis?
3. What are risk factors for this condition?

ANSWERS

1. The right hilum is enlarged due to adenopathy and perihilar consolidation. There is a right paratracheal soft tissue mass displacing the trachea to the left. The CT scan confirms large-volume right paratracheal lymphadenopathy.
2. Primary pulmonary tuberculosis.
3. The incidence of TB is increasing, particularly in inner city areas due to increasing immigrant populations from endemic areas, social deprivation and to the increasing prevalence of human immunodeficiency virus (HIV) in children.

RADIOLOGY HOT LIST

- The pattern of disease in childhood differs from the adult presentation (typically apical location without adenopathy). Focal consolidation (in any zone) is characteristically associated with paratracheal/hilar adenopathy (primary complex). The parenchymal lesion may not be apparent on the CXR.
- Lobar collapse may occur due to bronchial compression by mediastinal lymph nodes or secondary to endobronchial TB. Pleural effusion is present in 10%.
- The parenchymal lesion usually heals and calcifies within 12 months. However, haematogenous dissemination can cause miliary TB (fine nodular shadowing throughout the lungs).
- The X-ray appearances may continue to deteriorate while the child is receiving appropriate treatment.
- Always suspect TB if mediastinal lymphadenopathy is present in an at-risk patient.

CLINICAL HOT LIST

- The primary infection is usually respiratory due to the inhalation of *Mycobacterium tuberculosis*. Primary infection is usually asymptomatic but systemic symptoms may be present in 10%.
- Potential outcomes of primary infection are:

Development of immunity	Containment of infection by delayed hypersensitivity reaction and subsequent granuloma formation
Progressive primary TB	Inadequate immune response with local progression of disease
Miliary TB	Massive haematogenous dissemination
Post-primary TB	Endogenous reactivation or exogenous re-infection

FURTHER READING

Marais BJ, Donald PR, Gie RP et al. 2004: A proposed radiological classification of childhood intra-thoracic tuberculosis. *Pediatr Rad;* 34: 886–94.

Case 98

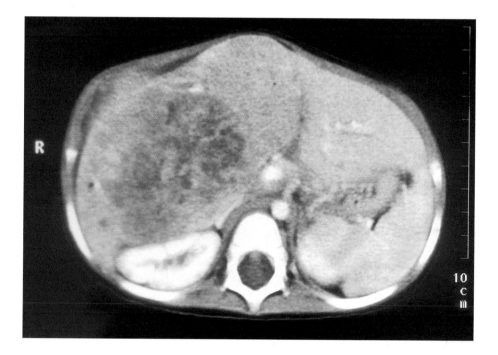

This 18-month-old girl presented to paediatric outpatients with a 2-month history of anorexia and weight loss. On examination there was a large mass in the right upper quadrant. Her serum alphafetoprotein (AFP) level was raised.

1. What abnormality is seen on the contrast-enhanced CT scan of the abdomen?
2. What is the most likely diagnosis?

ANSWERS

1. There is a large, ill-defined and mixed-attenuation mass within the right lobe of the liver. The left lobe is normal. The mass is displacing the surrounding organs but does not appear to invade them. The right anterior abdominal wall is distorted by the mass.
2. Hepatoblastoma.

RADIOLOGY HOT LIST

- Both hepatoblastoma and hepatocellular carcinoma appear as ill-defined, low-attenuation masses and demonstrate inhomogenous contrast enhancement. Biopsy is required for differentiation.
- CT and MRI are required to stage the tumour and assess its resectability.

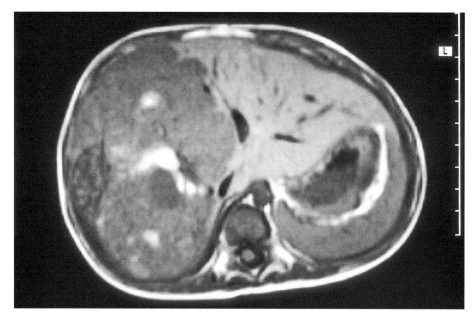

T1-weighted MRI showing hepatoblastoma.

- The differential diagnosis includes liver metastases (most commonly from neuroblastoma), and lymphoma.

CLINICAL HOT LIST

- Hepatic tumours represent 1% of childhood tumours (60% malignant, 40% benign haemangioma/hamartoma).
- Other abnormalities seen in hepatoblastoma include thrombocytosis, elevated AFP and abnormal liver enzymes. The serum AFP is useful in monitoring response to therapy and in screening those at risk, e.g. with Beckwith–Wiedemann.

	Hepatoblastoma	Hepatocellular carcinoma
Age	Under 5 years	5–15 years
Associations	Beckwith–Wiedemann, Wilms, hemihypertrophy	Hepatitis B and C, biliary atresia, α-1 antitrypsin deficiency, other causes of cirrhosis
Presentation	Abdominal mass; systemic features less common	Features of cirrhosis, splenomegaly, clubbing and pain; systemic manifestations more prominent
Management	Surgical excision, adjuvant chemotherapy	Chemotherapy and radiotherapy; less amenable to surgery

FURTHER READING

Von Schweinitz D. 2006: Management of liver tumors in childhood. *Semin Pediatr Surg;* 15: 17–24.
Donnelly LF, Bisset GS. 1998: Pediatric hepatic imaging. *Radiol Clin N Am;* 36: 413–27.

Case 99

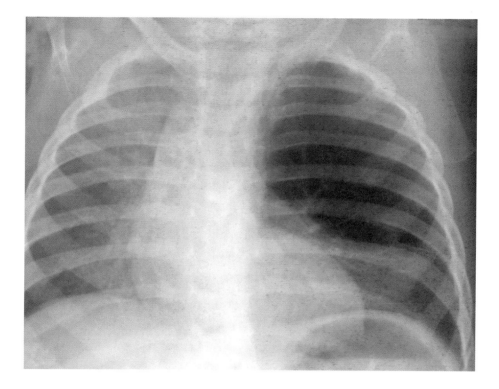

Following an uneventful pregnancy and labour, a term baby is noted to have a respiratory rate of 100 on his routine postnatal examination.

1. What do the chest radiograph show?
2. What is the diagnosis?

ANSWERS

1. The CXR shows a difference in transradiancy between the two sides of the chest, with increased lucency in the left upper and mid zones. The pulmonary vessels are attenuated in this area. There is minor mediastinal shift to the right, and there is volume loss in the left lower lobe.
2. Congenital lobar emphysema of the left upper lobe.

RADIOLOGY HOT LIST

- Overdistension of a lobe leads to hyperlucency of the affected lobe with collapse of adjacent lobes. Mediastinal shift may occur.
- Distribution of involvement: left upper lobe (40%), right middle lobe (30%), right upper lobe (20%).
- Initially, lung fluid may be trapped in the affected lobe due to impaired bronchial clearance, producing an opaque mass on the CXR. The classic radiographic findings occur as the fluid is replaced by air.
- CT can confirm the diagnosis and exclude the presence of either an extrinsic or endobronchial mass (such as a bronchogenic cyst) causing obstructive emphysema.

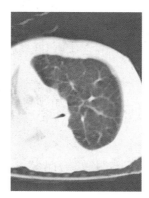

CT showing hyperinflation of the left upper lobe, which has reduced vascular markings.

CLINICAL HOT LIST

- Localized bronchomalacia or compression of a specific bronchus leads to overexpansion of that lobe secondary to air trapping. Additionally this compromises ventilation of the surrounding normal lung.
- 15% of cases are associated with congenital heart disease.
- 50% of cases present with neonatal respiratory distress, but delayed presentation in infancy with mild intermittent symptoms (respiratory and feeding difficulties) is well recognized.
- Surgical excision of the affected lobe is reserved for those who fail conservative management.
- There is increasing use of minimally invasive surgical technique, e.g. thoracoscopic procedures.

FURTHER READING

Paterson A. 2005: Imaging evaluation of congenital lung abnormalities in infants and children. *Radiol Clin N Am;* 43: 303–23.

Case 100

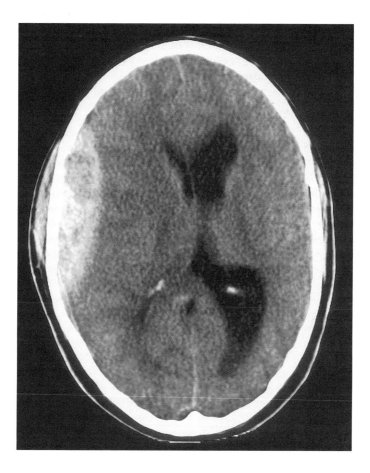

This 16-year-old male was brought to A & E following an assault. He was hit on the head with a snooker cue at his brother's 18th birthday party at the local pub. On arrival in A & E, he had signs of a left hemiparesis and soft tissue swelling over the right frontal region. He was intubated and ventilated prior to a CT scan.

1. What does the unenhanced scan show?
2. What is the diagnosis?

ANSWERS

1. There is a large convex high attenuation extracerebral collection in the right frontoparietal region. This is causing mass effect with midline shift, effacement of the right lateral ventricle and dilatation of the left lateral ventricle. There is associated right-sided extracranial soft tissue swelling.
2. A right extradural haematoma.

RADIOLOGY HOT LIST

- CT is the modality of choice for the detection of acute intracranial haemorrhage.
- An extradural haematoma is a collection of blood between the dura and the skull vault, usually associated with blunt trauma to the skull.
- The convex lenticular nature of the lesion is diagnostic of an extradural collection.
- There is an associated skull fracture in 40% of cases (up to 80% in adults).
- Additional findings may include extracranial soft tissue swelling, intracranial free air (suggesting a compound fracture), and intracerebral haemorrhage/contusions.

CLINICAL HOT LIST

- All children with an extradural collection warrant urgent neurosurgical referral.
- The classical history of a lucid interval is seen in < 50%.
- Prompt surgical evacuation is associated with excellent outcome, as there is rarely an underlying structural brain injury.

Case 101

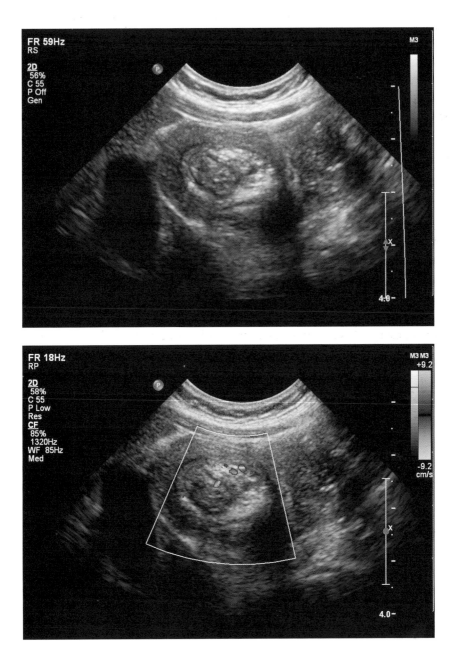

This 1-year-old boy presented with a sudden onset of screaming and vomiting. An ultrasound of the abdomen was performed.

1. Describe the USS appearances.
2. What is the diagnosis?

ANSWERS

1. The ultrasound shows an abnormal segment of bowel with a characteristic 'doughnut' sign. Blood flow is demonstrated within the bowel loop on colour Doppler imaging, due to mesenteric vessels within the lumen of the bowel.
2. Intussusception.

RADIOLOGY HOT LIST

- The value of the plain X-ray is debatable. It may be normal (25%), show a soft tissue mass (50%), and/or small bowel obstruction (25%). It may be useful in excluding other diagnoses.
- Ultrasound is almost always diagnostic with sensitivities and specificities approaching 100%. The classical appearance is of the 'doughnut' or pseudo-kidney sign. This is due to bowel loops and echogenic mesentery within the lumen of the intussusceptum. Absence of blood flow suggests bowel necrosis.
- The treatment of choice is by air reduction. The overall success rate is 70–85%. Reduction becomes increasingly difficult if the intussusception has been symptomatic for more than 48 hours. The contraindications are perforation, peritonitis and hypovolaemic shock, in which case the child should proceed to immediate surgery after resuscitation.

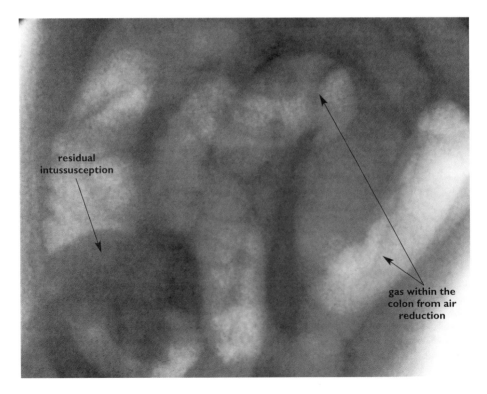

Air enema. The intussusception has been reduced into the caecum, where there is a residual soft tissue mass.

- Recurrence occurs in 6–10%, half within 48 hours of the initial reduction.

CLINICAL HOT LIST

- Invagination or prolapse of a segment of bowel into the lumen of adjacent intestine: ileocolic (75–95%) > ileoileal (4%) > colocolic.
- It is the commonest cause of acquired bowel obstruction in childhood. It is usually idiopathic, but a lead point (Meckel's diverticulum, lymphoma, polyp, duplication cyst, Henoch–Schönlein purpura) is present in 5%, usually in older children.
- The peak incidence is between 4 months and 2 years (< 10% of cases occur in children older than 3 years).
- Presentation is with acute onset of colicky abdominal pain, vomiting, redcurrant jelly stools and cardiovascular collapse. The typical history is of pallor, screaming and drawing up of the legs.
- Complications include vascular compromise (bowel infarction), bowel obstruction, and perforation and hypovolaemic shock.

FURTHER READING

Williams H. 2008: Imaging and intussusceptions. *Arch Dis Child Ed Pract;* 93: 30–6.

Case 102

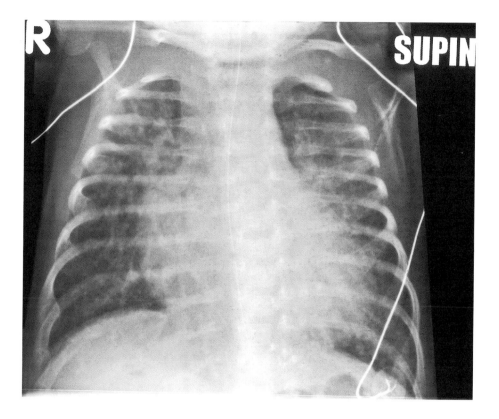

This 2-month-old boy with Down's syndrome has been short of breath at rest since birth. On examination he is not cyanosed.

1. What does the CXR show?
2. What is the most likely diagnosis?

ANSWERS

1. There is cardiomegaly with pulmonary plethora. No pleural effusion is seen.
2. Left-to-right shunt, most likely an atrioventricular septal defect (AVSD) in a child with Down's syndrome.

RADIOLOGY HOT LIST

- Cardiomegaly is defined as a cardiothoracic ratio (CTR) > 0.5 on a PA CXR. As most paediatric CXRs are taken AP, measuring the CTR is not always accurate. Gross enlargement is usually obvious.
- Causes of cardiomegaly include: congenital heart disease, congestive cardiac failure, pericardial effusion, myocarditis and cardiomyopathy.
- Acyanotic congenital heart disease with increased pulmonary vascularity is most commonly caused by a left-to-right shunt, which may occur at different anatomical sites.
- Causes of acyanotic congenital heart disease are:

Increased vascularity	Left-to-right shunts: ventriculoseptal defect (VSD), atrial septal defect (ASD), AVSD, patent ductus arteriosus
Normal/reduced vascularity	Pulmonary stenosis, aortic stenosis, coarctation of aorta

CLINICAL HOT LIST

- Congenital heart disease occurs in 40% of babies with Down's syndrome (50% will have an AVSD).
- Diagnosis may be antenatal. Postnatally this may present with a heart murmur or signs of cardiac failure.
- Definitive treatment is surgical repair—usually a single stage complete repair within the first 6 months of life. Occasionally pulmonary artery banding is used as a palliative procedure.
- Residual atrioventricular valve regurgitation or stenosis determines the long-term outlook, and the usual 10-year survival rate is > 80%.

FURTHER READING

Ferguson EC, Krishnamurthy R, Oldham SAA. 2007: Classic imaging signs of congenital cardiovascular abnormalities. *RadioGraphics;* 27: 1323–34.

Case 103

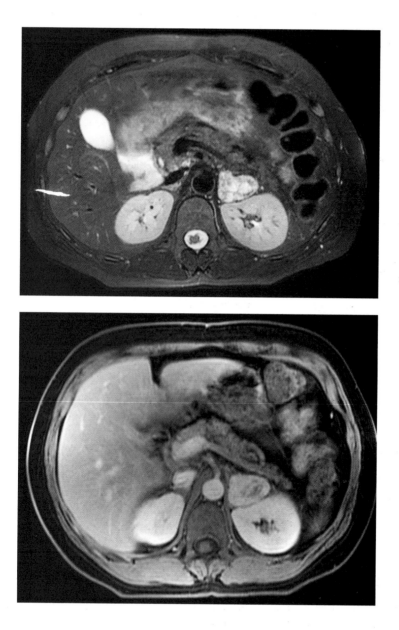

This 15-year-old girl suffers from episodes of sweating and palpitations. On examination she is tachycardic and hypertensive. She has raised serum and urinary catecholamines. An abdominal MRI scan has been performed.

1. What do the fat-saturated T2-weighted and the T1 post-contrast scans show?
2. What is the most likely diagnosis?
3. What other sequence will aid lesion characterization?

ANSWERS

1. There is a left adrenal mass lesion. This shows intense high signal on T2-weighted scans, and rapid contrast enhancement on T1-weighted scans. The appearances are suggestive of an adrenal tumour.
2. Phaeochromocytoma.
3. In-and-out of phase imaging, which will define the fat content of the lesion.

RADIOLOGY HOT LIST

- Phaeochromocytomas are often large tumours at presentation (> 3 cm) and may demonstrate areas of necrosis and haemorrhage.
- CT/MRI scans are used to identify and characterize adrenal lesions by assessing their fat content and enhancement characteristics. MIBG scans are more specific for phaeochromocytoma and are useful to detect extra-adrenal and metastatic disease.
- Adrenal adenomas are typically lipid-rich, so have a low CT value (< 10) on pre-contrast scans and lose signal on out-of-phase MR imaging. Other adrenal tumours usually have soft tissue density and no significant fat content.
- Benign adenomas show rapid uptake and washout of intravenous contrast. Scans are therefore acquired precontrast, at peak enhancement and in the delayed phase to assess the percentage washout.

CLINICAL HOT LIST

- These are very rare tumours arising from the catecholamine-producing chromaffin cells of the adrenal medulla. (An extra-adrenal paraganglioma is the equivalent arising from sympathetic or parasympathetic paraganglia). They may be benign or malignant.
- Strong genetic associations include: von Hippel–Lindau, multiple endocrine neoplasia type 2, neurofibromatosis type 1, familial paraganglioma.
- Presentation is very varied, from incidental finding on imaging to hypertensive crisis. Other symptoms include: sweating, flushing, palpitations, blurred vision, panic attacks, tremor and GI disturbance.
- 60% of affected individuals have hypertension.
- Diagnosis is by 24-hour urinary catecholamines and imaging.
- Management: surgery is curative for most but must be preceded by adequate pharmacological catecholamine blockade (α blockade before β blockade to prevent reflex tachycardia and rebound hypertension). Life-long follow up is required. Genetic review may be required for family members. Bilateral adrenalectomy necessitates steroid replacement.

FURTHER READING

Armstrong R, Sridhar M, Greenhalgh KL et al. 2008: Phaeochromocytoma in children. *Arch Dis Childhood;* 93: 899–904.

Blake MA, Holalkere NS, Boland GW. 2008: Imaging techniques for adrenal lesion characterization. *Radiol Clin N Am;* 46: 65–78.

Case 104

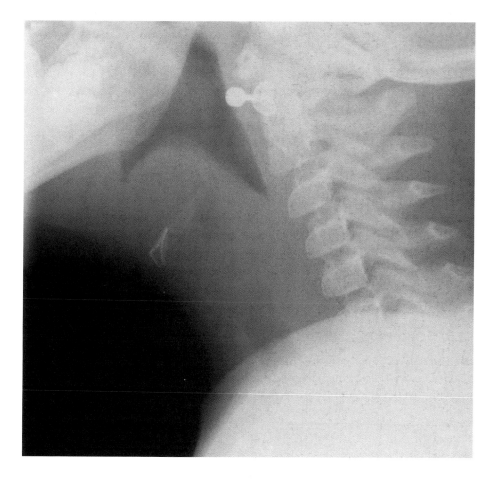

A 4-year-old girl has a fever and sore throat. On examination she is pyrexial (40°C) and drooling.

1. What abnormality does the lateral X-ray of the neck show?
2. What is the diagnosis?

ANSWERS

1. The epiglottis is enlarged and indistinct and encroaches on the pharynx. The upper airway is distended.
2. Acute epiglottitis.

RADIOLOGY HOT LIST

- Epiglottitis is a clinical diagnosis and a paediatric emergency. Radiographs are not required to make the diagnosis! If X-rays are performed, the child must be accompanied by a physician skilled in managing a paediatric airway—the risk of complete airway obstruction is very real.
- The normal epiglottis has a well-defined slender shape—in acute epiglottitis this shape is lost as the epiglottis becomes swollen, with swelling of the adjacent aryepiglottic folds, leading to airway obstruction.

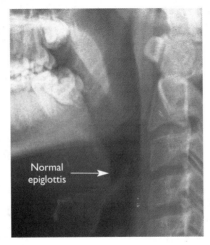

Lateral X-ray of neck showing normal epiglottis.

- The upper airway may be distended (airway obstruction) and the neck held in extension (to keep the airway patent).

CLINICAL HOT LIST

- It is due to a severe bacterial infection, usually occurring in 2–7-year-olds. It is now rare due to the *Haemophilus influenzae* B vaccination.
- Clinical presentation: sudden onset of sore throat and dysphagia, progressing to signs of upper airway obstruction in a febrile toxic child.
- Do not examine the child as this may provoke airway obstruction.
- No investigations are necessary prior to diagnostic laryngoscopy. Intubation or tracheostomy may be required; this must be undertaken in a controlled manner in theatre, with the most experienced anaesthetist and ENT surgeon available.
- Further management includes intravenous antibiotics and intensive care.

FURTHER READING

Majumdar S, Bateman NJ, Bull PD. 2006: Paediatric stridor. *Arch Dis Child Ed Pract;* 91: ep101–5.

Case 105

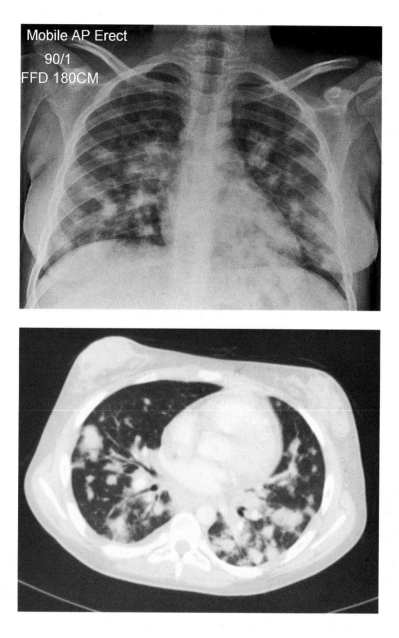

This 8-year-old boy has a cough and fever. He underwent a bone marrow transplant for thalassaemia 35 days ago. A CXR and chest CT scan have been performed.

1. What abnormality is seen on the CXR?
2. What does the CT scan of the chest show?
3. What is the most likely diagnosis?

ANSWERS

1. There are ill-defined infiltrates in the mid and lower zones of both lungs.
2. The CT shows multiple ill-defined pulmonary nodules, some of which have a 'ground-glass halo'.
3. Fungal chest infection in an immunocompromised host—most likely pulmonary aspergillosis. The differential diagnosis includes bacterial infection and pulmonary haemorrhage.

RADIOLOGY HOT LIST

- High-resolution chest CT is more sensitive than the plain radiograph, particularly in the early stages of infection.
- Radiographic findings in pulmonary aspergillosis include ill-defined nodules and consolidation.
- Angioinvasive aspergillosis characteristically shows a nodule or mass surrounded by a ground glass halo, representing haemorrhagic infarction.
- Cavitation is uncommon in the presence of neutropaenia but may occur during the recovery phase, usually when the neutrophil count is > 1.

CLINICAL HOT LIST

- Systemic fungal infections are opportunistic, affecting children with impaired immunity as a consequence of their condition or the treatment. Fungal infection is a common cause of pneumonia following BMT with an incidence of up to 70%.
- *Aspergillus* is the most common pathogen, and is commonly angioinvasive, causing haemorrhagic infarction, and may be airway invasive causing tracheobronchitis, bronchiectasis and pneumonia. Other fungi include candida, nocardia, mucormycosis and cryptococcus.
- Clinically patients present with fever, dyspnoea, pleuritic pain and a dry cough.
- Fungal infections are associated with a significant mortality rate of up to 90%.
- Treatment:
  1. Prevention—prophylaxis, e.g. fluaconazole.
  2. Infection—systemic antifungal, e.g. amphoteracin B.

FURTHER READING

Algar V, Novelli V. 2007: Infections in the immunocompromised host. *Paediatr Child Health;* 17: 132–6.

Case 106

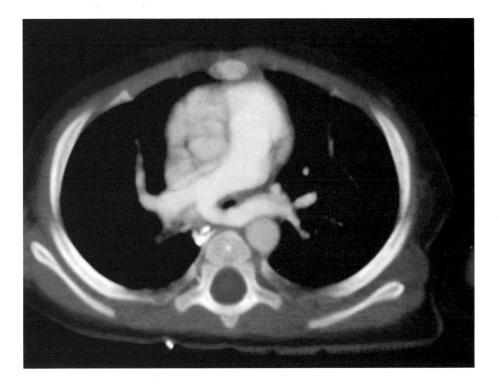

This 5-week-old baby has had stridor since birth. The child had a barium swallow followed by a CT chest scan.

1. What does the CT scan show?
2. What is the diagnosis?

ANSWERS

1. The left pulmonary artery has an anomalous origin and abnormal course, passing behind the trachea and creating a vascular sling. It passes in between the trachea and oesophagus, which contains an nasogastric (NG) tube. (Compare this to the normal anatomical orientation on page 15)
2. Aberrant left pulmonary artery forming a pulmonary artery sling.

RADIOLOGY HOT LIST

- A barium swallow is traditionally the first-line investigation of choice. The aberrant artery passes between the trachea and oesophagus, creating a characteristic anterior indentation of the oesophagus on the lateral view.
- Echocardiography usually confirms the aberrant position of the left pulmonary artery and may demonstrate other cardiac abnormalities (which are present in 50% of cases), most commonly atrial septal defects, patent ductus arteriosus and ventricular septal defects.
- CT cardiac angiography or cardiac MRI elegantly demonstrate the defect and associated cardiac and pulmonary anomalies, with the advantage of 3D reconstructions to aid surgical planning.

CLINICAL HOT LIST

- It is a rare defect that can cause death in the early months of life in severely affected infants.
- There is an anomalous origin of the left pulmonary artery from the posterior aspect of the right pulmonary artery, rather than the main pulmonary trunk. It loops around the trachea to reach the hilum of the left lung, creating a pulmonary artery sling.
- Compression of the trachea and right main bronchus results in upper airway symptoms. Other associated problems may include tracheomalacia and tracheal stenosis.
- Presentation is usually in the neonatal period with respiratory problems including stridor, wheeze, recurrent pneumonia and cyanosis.
- Medical care is supportive (ventilation, supplementary oxygen, antibiotics for infection) until the patient can undergo definitive surgical correction.
- Surgery involves division and re-anastamosis of the vessel. Postoperative mortality is often due to the high frequency of bronchial and tracheal abnormalities.

FURTHER READING

Yedururi S, Guillerman RP, Chung T et al. 2008: Multimodality imaging of tracheobronchial disorders in children. *RadioGraphics;* 28: e29, Published online.